Paediatrics

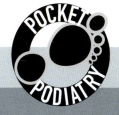

Angela Evans

PhD, GradDipSocSc, DipAppSc
University of South Australia, Australia

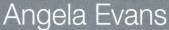

Series Editor
Ian Mathieson
BSc(Hons), PhD, MChS
Senior Lecturer, Wales Centre for Podiatric Studies,
University of Wales Institute, Cardiff, UK

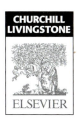

CHURCHILL
LIVINGSTONE

ELSEVIER

Edinburgh London New York Oxford Philadelphia St Louis Sydney Toronto 2010

CHURCHILL LIVINGSTONE
ELSEVIER

First published 2010, © Elsevier Limited. All rights reserved.

ISBN 978-0-7020-3031-4

British Library Cataloguing in Publication Data
A catalogue record for this book is available from the British Library

Library of Congress Cataloging in Publication Data
A catalog record for this book is available from the Library of Congress

Notice
Neither the Publisher nor the Author assume any responsibility for any loss or injury and/or damage to persons or property arising out of or related to any use of the material contained in this book. It is the responsibility of the treating practitioner, relying on independent expertise and knowledge of the patient, to determine the best treatment and method of application for the patient.

The Publisher

Printed in China

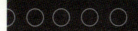

Contents

Foreword

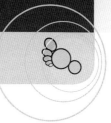

The publication of *Pocket Podiatry: Functional Anatomy* in summer 2009 carried a foreword that claimed it was the first of a series that would build into a comprehensive clinical guide. One text does not make a series however and, whilst basic clinical sciences are vital in that they underpin clinical practice, they cannot claim to be a true clinical discipline in their own right. Therefore the publication of *Pocket Podiatry: Paediatrics* not only represents the point at which the concept of a series comes to fruition but also the point at which it moves firmly into the clinical domain. We do so under the guidance of Dr. Angela Evans who writes about the clinical management of a patient group with whom most podiatrists have some contact but with whom relatively few truly specialise – children. Dr. Evans' text is highly informative – both academically and practically – and is written in a lucid, accessible style which conveys her real enthusiasm for and genuine insight to the subject. After dealing with basic issues including: an approach to the consultation; accounts of embryology and ontogeny; developmental biomechanics; and the development of gait, a series of specific conditions are discussed. These are diverse and include growing pains, clubfoot, metatarsus adductus, verrucae and the osteochondroses. A critical approach is adopted reflecting contemporary knowledge and evidence. As such this book provides invaluable information which will facilitate clinicians to develop an evidence based service. For example, details of various valid and reliable diagnostic aids are provided and chapters discussing specific conditions include evidence based treatment guidelines. I found this text both clinically informative and thoroughly engaging throughout. I am grateful to Dr. Evans for undertaking this project with such professionalism and commitment. I believe that you will find *Pocket Podiatry: Paediatrics* to be the genuinely informative and useful clinical companion it was designed to be.

Ian Mathieson
Cardiff, UK, 2009

Preface

This book is intended for undergraduate podiatry students but may well be of interest to a broader range of clinicians. Following Chapter 1, which addresses the clinical consultation with children, the book is basically constructed in three parts. Chapters 2–6 provide a necessary foundation to foot development and growth. Chapters 7–12 cover common paediatric foot/gait conditions and in addition to descriptive accounts, address clinical intervention from the perspective of an evidence-based medicine framework. It is important that intervention be justifiable and well thought out rather than applied because it is available or habitual. This is equally true of non-intervention. The third part, Chapters 13–15, is general in nature, with much of the content derived from my clinical experience. Here, I have attempted to merge currently available research evidence with clinical evidence, as reflects contemporary health care and from my worlds of both research and clinical practice.

The current research into children's foot posture should see contemporary research findings implemented within the realm of clinical practice. Specifically, the oft experienced dilemma of the flat-footed child can be more clearly understood, assessed and managed. The paediatric flat foot proforma is a helpful approach to directing concerns about children with flat feet. Having completed a doctoral thesis in the area of children's leg pain (growing pains) and foot posture, I am acutely aware, as both clinician and researcher, how important it is to have an effective merging of research findings into clinical practice if the public are to be recipients of 'best practice'.

This small text is in no way a definitive book nor exhaustive for the primary topic of paediatric podiatry. From the outset, I most strongly urge and encourage readers to regard this as a stepping off point of departure, from which many other paediatric, orthopaedic, medical, sociological and current research resources need also be consulted. Though covering a limited number and array of topics, this book will, I hope, prove useful nonetheless.

I am indeed grateful for the opportunity to have compiled this book and would like to thank Robert Edwards, my commissioning editor from Elsevier, for presenting this challenge. My grateful thanks are also due to my UK colleague Ian Mathieson, series editor, for his very helpful advice. I am indebted to Nicola Lally, Development Editor at Elsevier, Oxford, for her patience and assistance in seeing this book to its fruition. I wish to sincerely thank my colleagues, Margaret Carty and Michael Harding, for allowing me to use their children as photographic subjects and the many publishers who have granted permission for designated figure use. Additional thanks are due to Melissa McCaig, for preliminary draft proofreading and suggesting the chapter specific definition of terms.

Angela Margaret Evans
Adelaide, South Australia, 2009

Consulting with children

Introduction

Children are not a homogeneous group. In parallel to their physical development, children are simultaneously growing psychosocially. It is very important to recognize this fact when consulting with children, as they are not just scaled down adults. An appreciation of the stages of children's psychosocial development is both fascinating and necessary if one is to enjoy clinically successful consultations. By this, I mean a consultation which achieves its clinical end, be this assessment or treatment, and one which is a good experience for the child, parent/carer and clinician. To do this is both challenging and gratifying.

Milestones

Just as we have a set of expected milestones for physical development, those of us consulting with children require a similar knowledge of what is expected for ages and stages from a psychosocial perspective. Acknowledging that we are podiatrists, we require what may be termed a *working knowledge* of paediatric psychology and social science to enhance our clinical encounters with children of all ages. Table 1.1 outlines the main psychosocial stages of development, which it is useful to appreciate (Miller 1993).

Table 1.1 The development of psychosocial stages across the life span, according to Erikson*

Stage	Age	Concern	Clinical relevance
1	Birth to 1 year	Trust vs mistrust	Mother is usually primary; keep her close and all will be well. Be authentic and consistent with infants
2	2–3 years	Autonomy vs shame, doubt	Important for children to 'succeed' in the consult; help them to do the right thing by being clear and sensitive
3	4–5 years	Initiative vs guilt	Role models are important at this stage; be a good one
4	6 years to puberty	Industry vs inferiority	Children are keen to do things well; inform and acknowledge their efforts
5	Adolescence	Identity and repudiation vs identity diffusion	This is a potent stage – blooming and exciting for some, awkward and uncomfortable for others; be gentle (a grunt can be a socially acceptable whimper)
6	Young adult	Intimacy and solidarity vs isolation	Relationships are important; expect boyfriends/girlfriends to accompany, so include them
7	Middle adult	Generativity vs stagnation and self-absorption	Busy careers, often raising their own children; be clear and efficient (and on time)
8	Late adult	Integrity vs despair	The die is cast – positively or negatively. Be realistic and positive and prepared to listen for some real wisdom

*The development theorist Erik Erikson (a student of Freud) divided the life span into eight basic stages. An awareness of these stages is very useful and the first five apply directly to the paediatric domain. The clinical relevance column is sourced from this author's experience.

Do you like children? The crucial element of authenticity

I genuinely like children and enjoy their company. Children are extremely perceptive and can pick out a phony from the start. Such falsity arouses their suspicions that *all is not well* and induces fear and apprehension. This is quite justifiable and no amount of pandering and hollow words or gestures can fool these astute little people. The consultation will be, at best, an experience the child is pleased to see finish and at worst a frightening, traumatic event.

Some people just are not suited to working with children and it is painfully apparent. The lack of warmth, engagement and basic respect is almost palpable, as is the wariness, doubt and fear of the child, expressed more or less covertly by different children at different ages.

Thoughts as to why children cry

Basically, children cry when they are not happy. This can be for a variety of reasons and while as clinicians (as opposed to the children's parents/carers) we are not always able to identify the specific cause, we are able to consider the likely factors at play.

Children largely cry when they are:

- unwell
- tired
- anxious
- hungry
- scared.

Key *Concepts*

While distressing for everyone, a crying child gives ample opportunity for us to respond. There is nothing subtle about it and no excuse for missing the cue

However, there's crying and then there's *crying*. Personality, socialization, cultural background and fear will all play their part in how and when a child cries. While there are no hard and fast rules, I am often less concerned by a child who cries loudly and obviously as it is impossible to miss their distress and therefore easier to manage it. In general, it is a matter of slowing down and taking time to allay the child's fears. Children who have recently had their inoculations may not understand that this 'doctor' is just going to look at them walking. Play and explain, do not rush the pace (depending upon the age) and things will almost always settle down well. Children do not want to have a bad time any more than you do, but they are usually very honest about it. Respect their honesty, be honest in return and you will have a great time together. So often children are then reluctant to leave, which is a 'gold star' for you as a clinician, as is the overheard and unsolicited 'that was fun', or *'I like her'*, on the way out.

Children who are not crying may still be frightened

Please look out for these children, the stoic, reserved type who is trembling on the inside. As stated above, the child's personality, socialization, culture and fear will merge to influence how, where, when and with whom they express their feelings. It is the same for us. Our personality, socialization, culture and fear will influence how we perceive others and relate to them, especially with children.

Sensitivity and the 'three Fs'

This is a model that is very helpful when working with children, especially in the clinical setting where encounters are fairly brief, often unfamiliar and relatively intrusive.

Using the *three Fs* (Lally et al 1990) can help to avoid many otherwise likely pitfalls that can result in children being upset and mar the whole consultation. Especially valuable at the initial consultation, screening children's basic *modus operandi* (psychosocially) informs and directs aware adults. Recognizing and appreciating a child's fundamental style takes practice and it is important to realize that each *F* may be either overt or covert. The main tenets of the *three Fs* are:

1. Fearful

The child is basically wary and apprehensive, especially of new people, experiences and places. Anxiety is a dominant emotion and feeling. Eye contact with you may be brief or absent.

Overt

The child is obviously crying and clinging to a parent/carer. The pitch of the cry is scared, not angry (these subtle differences are easy to hear after a while).

Covert

The child puts on a brave face and complies. Their body language is 'louder' if you 'listen', e.g. blank expression, downcast eyes, and a stoop of the shoulders.

It is easy to mistake this quiet child for a flexible child and presume they are coping better than they are. Missing the cues from these 'easy' children can result in more overt fear and distress.

2. Flexible

These children are easy-going, cooperative and comfortable (for their age and situation). These children return your smile and maintain eye contact readily – some will stare you down, which can be disquieting until you get used to their genuine interest in you.

Overt

Flexible children will willingly comply with reasonable requests. They are not completely passive, but generally comfortable to work with you.

Covert

Children who hide their fear can be mistaken as being flexible. This is a pity, as too much is then expected from them and it can all come tumbling down.

Flexible children are easy to work with, as long as it is remembered that they are *children*. It is easy to overlook the needs of children who do not readily protest, which does not necessarily mean they are coping. Check to see if they are all right.

3. Feisty

From a cheerful whirlwind to a demanding inquirer, these children are usually difficult to miss. They are often busy, active and talkative (age dependent) and will very readily engage and want to know *precisely* what is going on. Give a clear account of what the consultation will entail and you will have a delightful time with these often entertaining children.

Overt

These children can be boisterous, loud and will introduce themselves and request you to do the same ('*What's your name?*', or '*I'm Emma and I'm four*' – be ready to reveal your age!).

Covert

Some of the incessant questioning from these children belies a latent element of fear as to what may be about to happen. It is important not to be seduced by a fierce or exuberant style. These children can masquerade as brave, but will crumble (loudly) if their fear is not recognized and allayed.

Courtesy

In addition to being authentic and sensitive with children, I believe that much of working with children comes down to being courteous and considerate.

Key Concepts

> The adult–child professional meeting is a very rich context and there are many mismatches to accommodate, some simple and apparent, others complex and unfamiliar. For in as much as children are smaller, younger and less powerful, it is the responsibility of the adult clinician to be hospitable, honest and professionally knowledgeable.

The absolute basics include:

- Greet the child and parent/carer.
- Introduce yourself by name to both the parent/carer and the child.
- Tell them what the consultation will involve.
- Run the *three Fs.*
- Observe and respond to the child's needs.
- Provide clear information.
- Offer to answer any questions.
- Thank the child and parent/carer for attending.
- Follow up, if arranged or agreed.

All of these aspects need to be age and circumstance appropriate and practice makes perfect. Some consultations are definitely easier than others; we are all human and we all have our good and bad days, children just as much as adults, but courtesy and consideration are paramount.

The concept of 'scaffolding'

According to the Russian psychologist Lev Vygotsky (1896–1934, my favourite contextual theorist, who has been called 'the Mozart of psychology' and who died of tuberculosis aged 37), humans are embedded in a social context and human behaviour cannot be understood independently of this context (Miller 1993).

Vygotsky extended the political and economic ideas of Marx and Engels to the field of psychology. His three main tenets were:

1. Humans transform themselves through labour and tool use, for example tools such as language shape children's thoughts.
2. Economic collectivism is paralleled by socially shared cognition, for example adults share their knowledge with children to advance their cognitive development.
3. Dialectical change, for example with development children constantly re-work their understandings to synthesize a position or stance (e.g. nature vs nurture).

Revolutionary for its time, Vygotsky's legacy maintains relevance in the clinical setting for those working with children. One of the fascinating and very useful concepts proposed by Vygotsky was the *zone of proximal development*.

Defined, Vygotsky's zone of proximal development is:

> *the distance between a child's actual developmental level and their higher level of potential development under the guidance of more capable peers or adult guidance.*

Accepting this concept, the more aware and skilled adult builds on the competencies a child already has and presents activities or tasks slightly beyond this level.

For example, an 8-year-old child presents with flat feet and ankle equinus. As a part of the management you include calf stretching exercises. This child (for our purposes named Tom) plays football and, if you ask, may already have an idea of how to do a basic calf stretch. If so, ask him to show you his method. Typically, the child's technique needs some improvement and this can be constructively achieved as follows:

Angela: 'Tom, can you show me how you do your calf stretches at footy please.'

Tom: ' Well, I mostly do it like this, sometimes, I think.'

(Tom places hands on wall, one foot behind other and leans in)

Angela: 'OK Tom, that's good, you already know what to do, but I'd just like to show you how to change a couple of things to make it work even better.'

(Angela demonstrates the parallel foot positioning, knee positioning, etc.)

Angela: 'Can you try that please and see if it works?'

Tom: 'Sure. Like this?'

(Tom does the stretch with back foot abducted)

Angela: 'Nearly … you just need to straighten up your back foot a bit more please.'

(Tom straightens his back foot)

Tom: 'Is that right?'

Angela: 'Great Tom, that's it. It's really important to do these stretches properly to get the most out of them for your footy. Do you think you can do this?'

Tom: 'Yeah, but I'll need someone to remind me.'

Tom's parent: 'I'll remind you Tom, in fact I'll do them with you and that will help both of us.'

By utilizing Tom's zone of proximal development, he has been able to extend his already established skills. By appreciating the child's existing competency, aware clinicians can help children to build beyond this and in doing so act as *scaffolding* between existing abilities and prospective skills. This approach acknowledges the child as an active participant in the whole learning process, a process in which adults prompt, hint and suggest rather than control. Vygotsky's sociocultural theory emphasizes that values, beliefs, customs and skills are transmitted (adult to child) to the next generation (Berk 1994). The importance of good adult role models cannot be overestimated.

Building rapport through parents/carers

The paediatric consultation is very different to the adult consultation. By definition, the child has a decision-making adult or adults with them, while adults generally make their own decisions and ask their own questions when consulting with you about their own issues. As a result, the level of communication is far more demanding, if it is to be effective.

Be practical. A mother has brought her 2-year-old child to see you as she is concerned about his knock knees; she has a 3-month-old baby at her breast, she is sleep deprived and she has forgotten the nappy bag – she is not going to remember everything or think deeply and does not need you to provide your full knowledge about the minutiae of knee development. Instead, offer the following:

- Make everyone comfortable (seat the mother, place the pram, respond to the children – book/toy/chair to engage the toddler).
- Get to the point of the visit and identify the concern or query.
- Involve the child to be examined (as far as possible) so as to extend the rapport you are building with the parent. This is a powerful part of the experience for young children. If they sense that Mummy/Daddy/Grandpa likes and trusts you, the child will too.
- Get used to the floor! It is often best to examine a toddler on the floor at their breastfeeding mother's side rather than interrupt a feed, insist on the use of your couch and effectively disturb everyone. This is not unprofessional, but realistic and considerate.
- Explain your relevant findings. This is not the time to display your full knowledge. Write down the findings in three to five clear points for

the mother to retain. This is very helpful when discussing findings with another parent/carer who was not present.

Special needs of special children

Prejudices, pride and past experiences may need to be addressed within our own frameworks if we are to optimize our consultations with children. To speak plainly, it is not very taxing to have to see a confident, well cared for, happy and attractive child who complies perfectly and immediately. For many clinicians, however, it can be far more challenging to see a child with an intellectual or physical disability who drools, screams or looks frankly odd. Clearly, this is a superficial and convenient example to present. However, many parents of children with special needs will relate the strong recoil with which they have on occasion been met, both from clinicians and from members of the public. Just think how much that must hurt and how unnecessary it is. I really encourage you to treat everyone the same, regardless of looks and ability. In my experience, it is embracing the full complement of human diversity that is so interesting and rewarding.

Engaging with ages and stages

While every child is an individual, developmentally there are sub-groups. From a clinician's perspective, I broadly nominate six age ranges to be aware of and to adapt accordingly. A summary of the psychosocial stages (ages 1–5) which occur in parallel is found in Table 1.1.

Babies: less than 6 months

These little bundles are easy to examine as long as some basics are attended to:

- Take a good history first. This gives you most of the information and guides and reduces the examination time.
- Keep them warm (leaving their hats on prevents heat loss).
- Let them feed (be sensitive if the mother is breastfeeding as not all mothers are comfortable to do so with you there).
- Do everything you can while they are asleep and wake them when necessary.
- Spend time letting them see you and hear your voice.
- Usually I examine babies on a parent's lap (Fig. 1.1A; if an older sibling is demanding the parent's attention and the baby is happy, I use my table – remembering always to hold on).

- Gradually touch and respond to their movements – remembering to be gentle.
- Wrap them up again, put them in their prams.
- Summarize your findings with parents.

Babies: 6–12 months

- Similar to above, but be aware that at this age infants are usually more wary of strangers (Fig. 1.1B).
- An age-appropriate book or toy can distract when you get to the examination, although personally I find that a basic description of what I am doing seems to entertain the child and simultaneously inform the parent (Fig. 1.2).
- This is quite an intimate space and the child is usually happy to be there if they sense a good rapport between you and their parent.
- Watching floor play is an important part of assessing this age group, so ensure the carpet is clean or that a floor rug is used.
- Again, assist with re-dressing if helpful.

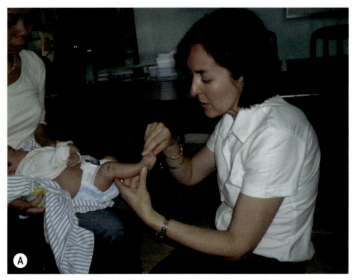

Figure 1.1 (A) Consulting with children can interrupt routines, so be flexible.

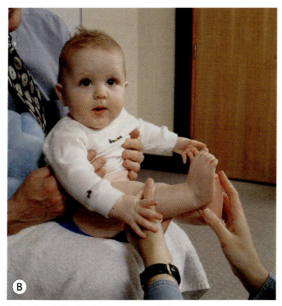

Figure 1.1 *Continued.* (B) Older babies are very alert.

New walkers

This is probably the prime time at which children will be brought to see you, as the feet and legs are suddenly more focal.

Children who are brought to see you because they are not walking need special attention, depending upon their age, history and your findings. Ensure you liaise with other health professionals as required and appreciate that walking age has a range (10–16 months).

- Ensure your rooms are safe for new walking explorers to visit.
- Never leave a mobile child unattended, even if the parents will.
- Children who are a little shy or overawed by the visit will often be happy to walk if you enlist the help of a parent in a 'passing' game, e.g. ask the parent to move a comfortable distance from the child and ask the child to walk to them. The parent can ask the child to get a toy from you or a strategically placed basket and then ask the child to bring it to them, place it somewhere or exchange it for something you may have (my pen is always a winning object). Little children love this game, often laughing delightedly as they walk,

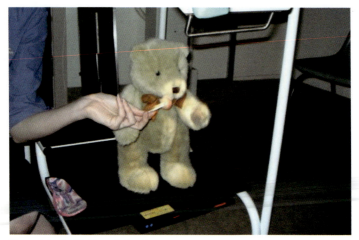

Figure 1.2 'Let Teddy go first… .'

giving you plenty of time to observe their postures and gait. Continuing the game seems to be more attractive than whether they are fully dressed or not and few protest when shoes, socks and trousers are removed by the parent.

- Review Chapter 5 regarding gait development and expected findings for age.
- Footwear advice is very relevant and important at this age so give specific advice about style, fit, foot growth and features. It is very helpful to have some shoe samples to show to parents (Ch. 14).

The *'terrific twos'* (but it can be a tough time for some)

Appreciating children's global development at this stage helps to understand the sometimes demanding encounters which may occur (Green 1994). As outlined in Table 1.1, children's psychosocial development has the issue of autonomy enmeshed within it at age 2 years. They are old enough to walk, talk and do many clever things by themselves but at the same time are easily shamed by mistakes and need a parent close at hand (but not too close). Speech is taking off and as a rule of thumb:

1-year-olds use single words, e.g. Daddy/Mummy/ball/teddy.

2-year-olds use word pairs, e.g. big car/Mummy here/thank you.

3-year-olds use three words together, e.g. I like you/Kate have it/you sit here.

4-year-olds form four or more word phrases, e.g. What are you doing?

The limitations of early speech can be visibly frustrating for children who know what they want and have to contend with adults doing otherwise. Trying to second-guess a 2-year-old can get rather fraught on both sides, but as adults we can try not to fan the flames by attempting to understand the child. It must be, and clearly is, maddening for children to have to deal with us sometimes.

It is usually easy to gain cooperation for gait evaluation, and while at this age children like to be independent, I never assume I will be able to examine them closely away from a parent's lap. Having said this, some children are looking forward to climbing up on to the table and feel duped if this is missed. Again it is important to look for and read the individual child's signals.

3–5-year-olds

Children of this age are really fun and rarely uncooperative without good reason. Make allowances for children who have had an unpleasant medical experience, as their fear will be running high, even if it manifests as belligerence or anger.

- Include the child in discussion and ask them the history questions they can answer, e.g.
  - How old are you?
  - Can you show me how you jump please?
  - Do you like climbing at the playground?
- Use age-appropriate language to explain the examination and cooperation is fairly assured, e.g.
  - Range of motion: 'Let's see which way your legs move.'
  - Muscle testing: 'Let's see how long your muscles are.' 'You tell me when it feels tight.'
- I often ask the child to hold my pen or reflex hammer when I am examining, as it involves/distracts them and gives me an extra hand.

Primary school (5–12 years)

These children are again generally easy to work with and are interested in learning about their feet and often quite enamoured with medical terms, e.g. *calcaneal apophysitis*. It is comforting for them to hear that other children have similar situations.

The older end of this age group are often interested in cause and effect and readily follow a well laid out treatment plan (with parental support).

Empowering children to be able to assist the process is useful and most parents are keen to share the responsibility with their upper primary school-aged children.

This age group is progressively literate and can be very interested and motivated by well-chosen educational brochures and websites, especially if you take the time to personalize the areas of relevance for them.

Secondary school (12–17 years)

Many of these children attend (subsequent) appointments by themselves or with a parent who stays in the waiting room. This is an obvious cue about the level of independence and family dynamics. (Your workplace may require children to be accompanied by a parent or caregiver.) If you need to speak to the parent, ask the child first, so as not to usurp their role. If the parent is not present and you need to speak with them, tell the child that you will call their parent to discuss the situation. It can be demeaning for children to be 'talked around' without their knowledge and does nothing to establish trust or respect in the teen–clinician relationship (Berne & Savary 1993).

Watch your language! In trying to relate to this age group it is very 'uncool' for an adult to try to be 'cool'. Instead, retreat to the safe zone of authenticity. Your credibility will be assured and it is a basic pre-requisite for trust at all ages and fundamental for *esprit de corps.*

References

Berk LE 1994 Child development, 3rd edn. Allyn and Bacon, Needhan Heights, MA

Berne PH, Savary LM 1993 Building self-esteem in children. Continuum Publishing, New York

Green C 1994 Toddler taming, 3rd edn. Doubleday, Sydney

Lally JR, Mangione PL, Signer S 1990 Flexible, fearful, or feisty: the different temperaments of infants and toddlers [videotape]. Program for Infant/Toddler Caregivers, developed collaboratively by the California Department of Education and WestEd, San Francisco

Miller PH 1993 Theories of developmental psychology, 3rd edn. WH Freeman, New York

Embryology and fetal development

Definition of embryology and fetal development

The period of in utero development from conception to the eighth gestational week (of the embryo) and henceforth, until birth (of the fetus).

Introduction

As podiatrists, it is important to have a fundamental understanding of the physical development of the foot and leg from conception to birth and beyond. This chapter presents a very basic précis of the physiological and neurological developments that occur to influence the eventual lower limb. It is wise to regard this chapter as a working guide, and your are advised to expand your knowledge by looking at the work listed in 'Further reading'.

This chapter will address the development of the foot during the embryonic and fetal periods and summarizes the expected morphology which accompanies full-term (versus pre-term) gestation. Many of the pathologies later encountered have their origins in aberrant development within the embryonic period and beyond.

Embryonic period

The embryonic period includes the germinal period (conception + 14 days), but technically begins at the third week post-conception and ends at the end of week 8 (Payne & Isaacs 2008).

From the time of fertilization of the ovum, myriad changes occur to convert the pre-lower limb buds to the eventual individual foot bones which are, in the main, present at the end of gestation. The embryonic period is defined as the first seven post-ovulatory weeks (Tachdjian 1997) and is divided into 23 stages or horizons, each of which corresponds to a developmental stage of the embryo (as described by Streeter, Carnegie, see Further reading; Sarrafian 1993). These stages are based on the external and/or internal morphological development of the embryo, rather than age or size (Fig. 2.1).

The embryonic cell mass or zygote divides and differentiates to form:

- *Ectoderm*: forms epidermis, sensory receptors and nervous tissues
- *Mesoderm*: forms skeletal, connective, muscle and blood tissues
- *Endoderm*: inner layer which forms the respiratory and gastrointestinal tract linings.

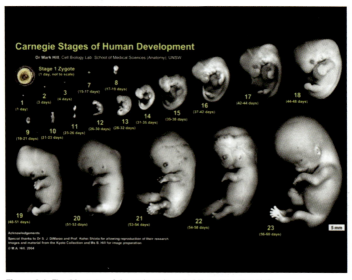

Figure 2.1 The 23 stages of the embryonic period (from 0 to 7 weeks).

Teratogens

The embryonic period is when the placenta, umbilical cord and amniotic fluid develop. During this period, the embryo is most susceptible to teratogens as the mother's blood is shared with the developing embryo. Thalidomide, a tranquillizing drug, is an infamous example of teratogen exposure adversely affecting development, but common recreational drug use is also implicated, e.g. alcohol, tobacco, cannabis, cocaine (Payne & Isaacs 2008).

Specific anomalies associated with recreational drug use include:

Alcohol
- Growth retardation, craniofacial abnormalities, CNS dysfunction.
- Fetal alcohol syndome (FAS) represents a cluster of birth defects due to prenatal alcohol exposure and includes:
  - ADHD (attention deficit, hyperactivity disorder)
  - mental retardation
  - altered facial features
  - decreased physical growth
  - reduced brain growth and lower IQ.
- Less severe problems are termed alcohol-related neurodevelopmental disorders (ARNDs) and include:
  - slow motor development
  - speech problems
  - clumsiness.

The point needs to be made that there is no safe level of maternal alcohol consumption during pregnancy and as little as one daily drink has been associated with retarded growth (Payne & Isaacs 2008).

Tobacco
- The main issues associated with tobacco use during pregnancy are increased miscarriage rate, increased infant mortality, lower birth weight and twice the incidence of sudden infant death syndrome (SIDS) (Machaalani & Waters 2008). Both carbon monoxide and nicotine (two of the many tobacco by-products) contribute to fetal hypoxia.
- Postnatally, children who live in homes with prevalent smoking are more likely to exhibit respiratory diseases.

Cannabis
- While cannabis use in pregnancy has been associated with lower birth weight, there is less stringent evidence for deleterious effects than for tobacco and alcohol where the evidence is conclusive.

However, it is known that THC (11-hydroxy-delta-9-tetrahydrocannabinol), the most active mind-altering ingredient, does cross the placenta and can accumulate in the fetus. Hence abstinence of cannabis use during pregnancy is advised (Klonoff-Cohen & Lam-Kruglick 2001).

Cocaine

- Whether smoked, snorted or injected the effects of cocaine are known to be among those most dangerous to the unborn baby. Premature gestational term (with all associated hazards) is increased by approximately 25% and fetal brain damage is at least four times higher than normal. As infants, cocaine-damaged babies are often both unresponsive and irritable, making care difficult and neglect or abuse more likely (Gingras et al 2004).

Common other drugs, maternal diseases and some genetic factors are summarized in Table 2.1.

The sixth, seventh and eighth embryonic weeks are those most associated with the development of lower limb defects (Drennan 1992, Tachdjian 1985) and most major congenital abnormalities occur within the eight embryonic weeks (Payne & Isaacs 2008).

Development of the foot

The foot is derived from condensed mesenchyme (from mesoderm) projecting through the ectoderm to form the template or anlage of the foot. There are three main stages to the forming of the skeleton:

- Mesenchymal
- Cartilaginous
- Osseous.

The mesenchyme differentiates to form metatarsals, phalanges and the tarsus. Cartilage (or its precursor called procartilage) appears within the areas of condensed mesenchyme and forms a chondrified anlage. Chondrification is largely complete by the end of the embryonic period. Vascular infiltration occurs initially in the talus from the arteries within the sinus tarsi (Tachdjian 1985). The vascular supply then spreads to supply the calcaneus, navicular, cuboid, cuneiforms, metatarsals and phalanges and signals the nearing of ossification. Endochondral ossification then ensues and in a general sense progresses from forefoot to rearfoot, with the distal phalanx of the great toe being the first foot bone to ossify. The calcaneus is the first tarsal bone to ossify and the navicular the last, varying between 2 and 5 years post-birth (Evans et al 2003). The cuboid

Table 2.1 Common drugs, maternal diseases and genetic factors which may affect fetal development

Drug	Use	Possible risks for fetus
Prescribed drugs		
Anticoagulants	Blood clots	Miscarriage CNS, eye defects
Antibiotics	Infections	Altered teeth development
Anticonvulsants	Seizures	Neural tube defects Hand, face defects Mental retardation
Over-the-counter drugs		
Aspirin	Pain, inflammation	Prolonged labour Increased mother's bleeding/bleeding within baby's skull during birth
Ibuprofen	Anti-inflammatory	Oligohyramnios (high use)
Maternal diseases		
Diabetes		Macrosomia, childhood obesity CNS, spina bifida Heart defects
HIV (human immunodeficiency virus)	**1.** In utero: mother to fetus **2.** Delivery: baby infected with blood/fluids **3.** Breast milk: zidovudine has reduced HIV in susceptible cases to approx. 5%	Survival approx. 24 months 90% symptoms by 4 years Few live past 13 years (AIDS)
Rubella (German measles)	Congenital rubella syndrome	Deafness (80% of cases) Hepatitis, pneumonia Glaucoma, cataracts Growth/mental retardation
Genetic factors		
	Chromosome 21 (trisomy)	Down's syndrome
	Chromosome 15	Angelman syndrome Prader–Willi syndrome Marfan's syndrome
	Chromosome 17	Charcot-Marie-Tooth (1A)
	Chromosome 2 (deletion)	Talipes equinovarus

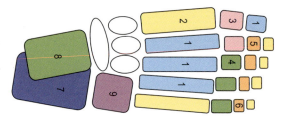

Figure 2.2 Ossification sequences.

ossifies at 37 weeks' gestation and is often used as a marker for fetal maturity. The chronological sequence of fetal foot ossification is shown in Figure 2.2.

The developing nervous system is evidenced in the third embryonic week when the ectoderm thickens to form the neural plate, which in turn gives rise to the neural groove and crest. Folding of the neural groove forms the neural tube which fuses and elongates in the fourth embryonic week to form the spinal cord. Much differentiation of the neural crest occurs to form various sensory and autonomic ganglia. While rapid growth of the brain occurs mid-gestation, 85% of brain growth occurs after birth (Shepherd 1995). A primitive lumbosacral plexus is formed by 5 weeks with the femoral, obturator, tibial and common peroneal nerves branching to their respective areas of the limb bud (Bareither 1995).

The lower limb buds first appear between three and five embryonic weeks, slightly later than the upper limb buds, and are positioned slightly lateral to the fifth lumbar and first sacral myotomes (the lumbar-sacral plexus bifurcates into the dorsal and ventral branches to supply extensor and flexor muscles, respectively) (Cusick 1990, Sarrafian 1993). Once begun, the development of the lower limb is fast, with discernible changes every 2 days. Prior to the fifth embryonic week the three regions corresponding to thigh, leg and foot are visible (Sarrafian 1993).

At 6 weeks the limbs are perpendicular to the body and laterally rotated at 90°, appearing as paddles or flippers. The foot is in full equinus and inverted. The plantar surfaces of the feet face each other in what has been termed a 'praying' position. Bud webbing begins to notch and regress to form digits. Webbed feet or syndactyly may result from incomplete regression of the limb bud webbing.

At 7 weeks the muscles of gastrocnemius and soleus are apparent with myogenous zones for the other flexors, extensors and peroneals present but ill-defined. The main nerves have branched to supply and innervate these future muscle groups (Bareither 1995).

Key *Concepts*

Many congenital deformities of the foot occur before the seventh embryonic week, at which point structural/skeletal components are determined (Tachdjian 1985). Limb malformations are frequently associated with other organ defects and often form part of a systemic syndrome.

Polydactyly, a common deformity in which there are more than five toes, results as part of altered genetic programming of limb development. It has long been recognized that polydactyly often indicates more general issues and before prenatal ultrasound screening was frequently the first question asked when a child was born (Talamillo et al 2005) (Fig. 2.3A, B).

Fetal period

Defined as the period between week 8 and term (40 weeks' gestation), the fetal period finds the developing foot in marked equinus, supinated and adducted. Muscles, vessels and nerves are differentiated and the digits are now distinct. The third toe is initially the longest in the very young embryo, to be overtaken by the second. The first toe usually, but not always, overtakes the length of the second. Similarly, the third metatarsal is initially the longest but is surpassed by the second metatarsal in fetal weeks 16–20. From week 24 onwards the second metatarsal becomes longer than the first, with the first occasionally shorter than the third (Sarrafian 1993, Tachdjian 1985).

At 9 weeks the calcaneus moves from adjacent to the talus to plantar to the talus. This forms the subtalar joint. The tibia and fibula begin to form an ankle mortise around the forming talar dome. The first metatarsal base articulates with the medial cuneiform, resulting in a wide intermetatarsal angle so that the first metatarsal and great toe are adducted. The distal phalanx of the great toe is the first bone to ossify.

Between weeks 10 and 12 the foot begins to dorsiflex at the ankle from its position of extreme equinus. The fetus is 75 mm long at 12 weeks and begins to move its legs and has clenched fists. The inverted position of the foot continues with torsion of both the head and the neck of talus and also the distal calcaneus.

At this stage the tibia and fibula are equal in length for the last time, with the fibular length increasing from now onwards. Pre-form nail tissue appears.

At 16 weeks the feet evert due to torsional changes in the talus and calcaneus. The medial longitudinal arch develops and true, layered skin

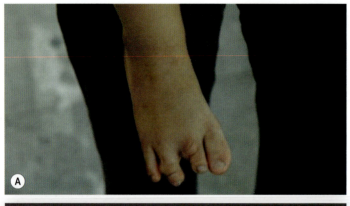

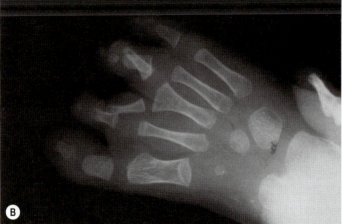

Figure 2.3 (A) Covert polydactyly where six phalanges (seen on X-ray) present clinically as four toes.
(B) Note the larger third metatarsal head which gives rise to two phalanges.

begins. This movement of eversion and dorsiflexion of the foot continues until birth and postnatally until approximately 6 years. The arms are now longer than the legs, a parameter that equalizes by 2 years and from then reverses.

At 18 weeks the fetus is 15 cm in length. By 21 weeks the calcaneus ossifies and is the first tarsal bone to do so (Fig. 2.4). At 22 weeks the

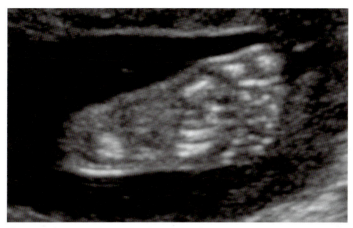

Figure 2.4 Sonographic image of the in utero fetal foot at 22 weeks. The calcaneus can be clearly seen as the first tarsal bone to have ossified.

fetus is 30 cm long and has hair on its head. The nails are now present. At 24 weeks the ossification centre of the talus appears.

From approximately 26 weeks the fetal spine becomes increasingly flexed from cervical to sacral vertebrae. At 37 weeks the cuboid ossifies and is used as an indicator of fetal maturity, in conjunction with ear cartilage.

Term versus pre-term gestation

Normal or 'full-term' human gestation is 40 weeks or between 266 and 280 days. The normal fetal term weight is about 3500 g (7.5 lb) and length about 50 cm (19.7 inches). The normal fetal posture is one of flexion, the fetus having been increasingly space confined as pregnancy progressed.

Pre-term or 'premature' infants display many characteristics which see them differ from their full-term counterparts. By definition and convention, babies born prior to 37 weeks' gestation are 'pre-term' but any of the traits displayed in Table 2.2 are also signs of immaturity. The general appearance of the infant includes a relatively large head with small, red, wrinkled face. The body is lean and wrinkly (yet to be 'filled out') and both the limbs and the nails are short. The abdomen is prominent and the body hair (lanugo) is increased (Fig. 2.5A, B).

There is a demonstrated high frequency of minor neuromotor dysfunctions (MNDs) at age 5 years associated with prematurity. According to

Table 2.2 Features of pre-term babies (<37 weeks' gestation)

Clinical feature	Related measure	Comment
Birth weight	<2500 g (5.5 lb)	Mothers with diabetes may have heavier premature babies Now regarded as 'low birth weight' (LBW) and babies <1500 g are termed 'very low birth weight' (VLBW). Babies <500 g are classified as 'extremely low birth weight' (ELBW)
Birth length	<30 cm (11.8 in)	
Hypotonia – 'floppy baby'	• Scarf sign • Knee extension • Ventral suspension • Extended posture • Poor recoil response	• Hand can be moved past opposite shoulder with ease • Limp head and limbs: cannot overcome gravity • Lies flat when placed supine rather than flexed
Ankle range	• Reduced ankle dorsiflexion available	• Due to underdeveloped joints
Weak reflexes	• Moro • Suck • Grasp • Walking	
Epiphyses	• Femoral (36 weeks) and tibial (37 weeks)	Absence of the distal femoral and proximal tibial epiphyses. Presence/absence of these epiphyses is a reliable newborn maturity indicator
Cuboid absence	• Normally present at 37 weeks	Presence/absence is a reliable newborn maturity indicator
Ear cartilage absence	• Normally occurs at 36 weeks	Presence/absence is a reliable newborn maturity indicator

gestational age, associations with behavioural and learning difficulties are related findings. The high rate of MNDs and their association with an increased risk for learning difficulties justifies screening in instances of even moderate prematurity (Arnaud et al 2007).

Low birth weight risks

Infants who are born pre-term or secondary to intrauterine growth restriction account for many and increased postnatal problems and subsequent

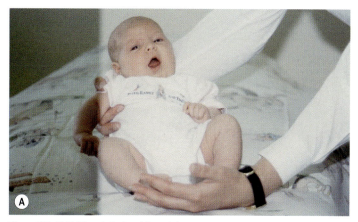

Figure 2.5 (A) Full-term baby (aged 5 weeks).

healthcare costs (Goldenberg & Culhane 2007). Low birth weight (LBW) in general places the infant at greater risk of later adult chronic medical conditions, such as lung disease (Lipsett et al 2006), diabetes (Akcakus et al 2006, Jensen et al 2007), hypertension and heart disease (Goldenberg & Culhane 2007, Jensen et al 2007). Not all low birth weight babies are premature; some result from intrauterine deprivation and are termed small for gestational age (SGA). The clinical outcomes for LBW associated with intrauterine impoverishment often include mental retardation, whereas LBW associated with prematurity is clinically linked to diplegia (cerebral palsy) (Payne & Isaacs 2008) (see Table 2.2).

Apgar scores

The Apgar score is a scaled rating system developed by Dr Virginia Apgar in the 1950s which assesses the newborn infant's need for life support. It is scored out of 10 and based on the sum of two points for each of the systems, as shown in Table 2.3.

This assessment of the newborn infant is made at 1 minute post-birth and again after 5 minutes. Normal scores are 7 or greater at 1 minute and 8 or more at 5 minutes. An Apgar score of 7 or more indicates that the baby does not require assistance; scores between 6 and 4 indicate that help is needed; scores 3 or less signal the urgent need for resuscitation (Thomson 1993). There is strong association between Apgar scores

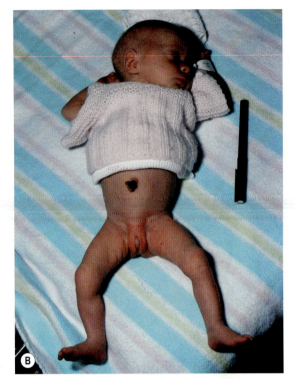

Figure 2.5 *Continued.* (B) Pre-term baby (born at 33 weeks' gestation). Note the residual physiologic flexion and 'filled out' appearance of the full-term baby in comparison to the extension and lean body mass of the pre-term baby (and the comparative size of a pen).

Table 2.3 Apgar scoring system*

Score	Heart rate	Respiratory effort	Muscle tone	Reflexes	Colour
0	Absent	Not crying	Flaccid	None	White or blue
1	<100/min	Shallow cry	Extremities flexed	Grimace	Pink body, blue extremities
2	>100/min	Strong cry	Flexed limbs and moving	Coughs	Fully pink

*Apgar score indicates the need for life-support at birth. Babies are scored for each of the five criteria at 1 and 5 minutes post-birth. Scores of ≥7–8 are normal.

of 0–3 at both 1 and 5 minutes with mortality and cerebral palsy (Moster et al 2001).

Children with low Apgar scores and subsequent signs of cerebral depression (but who do not develop cerebral palsy) may still have an increased risk of developing a range of neuro-developmental impairments and learning difficulties (Moster et al 2002).

Growth

Growth charts have become primary global child health instruments but until recently have not linked birth and postnatal growth values continuously. Swedish researchers have now resolved this issue by producing a single standard that bridges size at birth with postnatal growth. Importantly, the mean and 10th centile values compare similarly with reference values from Australia, UK, USA and Norway. The resulting charts are gender-specific and show continuous normal growth patterns from the 24th gestational week to 24 months of age (Niklasson & Albertsson-Wikland 2008). This reference tool should enable easier detection of growth deviations, which are so important in monitoring individual infant development.

Foot growth

Foot growth per se is only possible after the embryo reaches horizon 21, when the crown to rump length measures 24 mm. The foot grows quite quickly until the eighth week, then slows until week 14, grows rapidly to week 26 and then slows until term. From the 14th week the average weekly foot growth is 3 mm. The average length of the foot at 40 weeks' gestation (term) is 7.6 cm (range 7.1–8.7 cm) (Sarrafian 1993).

Foot growth continues to be very rapid until 5 years of age. The growth rate is reduced between age 5 and skeletal maturity of the feet, which occurs on average by age 12 years in girls and by age 14 years in boys (Tachdjian 1997). Figure 2.6 depicts the rates of fetal and foot growth in parallel.

Newborn feet that have a wider space between first and second toes and/or a plantar crease between first and second metatarsals may be associated with Down's syndrome (Thomson 1993). Clubfeet (talipes equinovarus) are usually readily identified. The best initial treatment is the Ponseti method which is now universally accepted as the first choice approach and 'gold standard' treatment (Morecuende et al 2004; Ponseti et al 2003, 2006). The Ponseti method is discussed in Chapter 8.

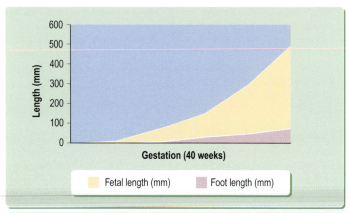

Figure 2.6 Foot and fetal lengths over 40 weeks.

Table 2.4 Attitudes of the foot and leg at birth and during normal development

Anatomical part	Position at birth	Positional change with growth
Calcaneus	Varus	Reducing until 6 years
Hip, knee and ankle	Laterally rotated	Reduces by 6 years
Tibia	0–6° lateral torsion	Increases to 18–23° by 6 years
Femoral neck inclination	Coxa valga (135° to femoral shaft)	Reduces by puberty/adulthood
Spine	Kyphotic	Develops cervical and lumbar lordoses
Pelvis	Shallow acetabulae which are inclined upward	Acetabulae deepen and angular postion 'declines'
Hip	In a position of flexion, abduction and lateral rotation	Develops extension Adduction and lateral rotation reduce

The foot and lower limb at birth

Table 2.4 illustrates the attitudes of the foot and leg at birth and the subsequent changes which occur with growth and development in readiness for bipedal weight-bearing and gait just 12 months away.

From birth until 6–7 years of age, there are a number of changes in alignment and mobility which occur due to the combination of osseous modelling and growth. Normal neuromotor development is crucial to the dynamic changes which need to occur to convert the very plastic infant

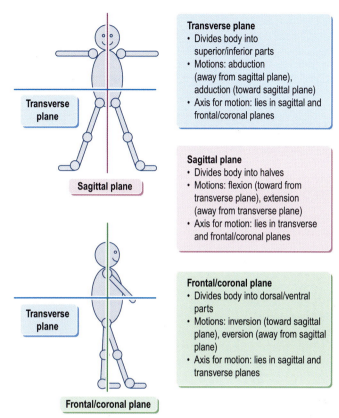

Transverse plane
- Divides body into superior/inferior parts
- Motions: abduction (away from sagittal plane), adduction (toward sagittal plane)
- Axis for motion: lies in sagittal and frontal/coronal planes

Sagittal plane
- Divides body into halves
- Motions: flexion (toward from transverse plane), extension (away from transverse plane)
- Axis for motion: lies in transverse and frontal/coronal planes

Frontal/coronal plane
- Divides body into dorsal/ventral parts
- Motions: inversion (toward sagittal plane), eversion (away from sagittal plane)
- Axis for motion: lies in sagittal and transverse planes

Figure 2.7 Definition of terms for planes of motion and related positions.

skeleton to a more static form. Normal developmental arrest may be gross or subtle and results in many of the later foot problems which the podiatrist must appreciate. Knowledge of the early development of the lower limb allows the astute practitioner to more ably explore the aetiology of presenting conditions in children and adults.

Summary

When the podiatrist meets the child's foot they are presented with the results of intricate, complex and rapid growth and development. An appreciation of this formation is clearly advantageous and necessary in recognizing normal and abnormal findings in the paediatric foot and leg post-birth. It is my experience that a basic working knowledge of embryology and fetal development serves not only diagnostically but also in building a sensitive rapport with the infant, child and parents as one acknowledges this most wondrous growth.

See Figure 2.7 for a definition of terms for planes of motion and related positions.

References

Akcakus M, Koklu E, Kurtoglu S et al 2006 The relationship among intrauterine growth, insulinlike growth factor 1 (IGF-1), IGF-binding protein-3, and bone mineral status in newborn infants. American Journal of Perinatology 23(8):473–480

Arnaud C, Daubisse-Marliac L, White-Koning M et al 2007 Prevalence and associated factors of minor neuromotor dysfunctions at age 5 years in prematurely born children: the EPIPAGE Study. Archives of Pediatrics and Adolescent Medicine 161(11):1053–1061

Bareither D 1995 Prenatal development of the foot and ankle. Journal of the American Podiatric Medical Association 85(12):753–764

Cusick BD 1990 Progressive casting and splinting for lower extremity deformities in children with neuromotor dysfunction. Therapy Skill Builders, Arizona

Drennan JC 1992 The child's foot and ankle. Raven Press, New York

Evans AM, Scutter S, Iasiello H 2003 Sonographic investigation of the paediatric navicular – an exploratory study in four year old children. Journal of Diagnostic Medical Sonography 19(4):217–221

Gingras JL, Mitchell EA, Grattan KJ 2004 Effects of maternal cigarette smoking and cocaine use in pregnancy on fetal response to vibroacoustic stimulation and habituation. Acta Paediatrica 93(11):1479–1485

Goldenberg RL, Culhane JF 2007 Low birth weight in the United States. American Journal of Clinical Nutrition 85(2):584S–590S

Jensen CB, Storgaard H, Madsbad S et al 2007 Altered skeletal muscle fiber composition and size precede whole-body insulin resistance in young men with low birth weight. Journal of Clinical Endocrinology and Metabolism 92(4):1530–1534

Klonoff-Cohen H, Lam-Kruglick P 2001 Maternal and paternal recreational drug use and sudden infant death syndrome. Archives of Pediatrics and Adolescent Medicine 155(7):765–770

Lipsett J, Tamblyn M, Madigan K et al 2006 Restricted fetal growth and lung development: a morphometric analysis of pulmonary structure. Pediatric Pulmonology 41(12):1138–1145

Machaalani R, Waters KA 2008 Neuronal cell death in the sudden infant death syndrome brainstem and associations with risk factors. Brain 131(1):218–228

Morecuende JA, Dolan LA, Dietz FR et al 2004 Radical reduction in the rate of extensive corrective surgery for clubfoot using the Ponseti method. Pediatrics 113(2):376–380

Moster D, Lie RT, Isaacs LD et al 2001 The association of Apgar score with subsequent death and cerebral palsy: a population-based study in term infants. Journal of Pediatrics 138(6):798–803

Moster D, Lie RT, Markestad T 2002 Joint association of Apgar scores and early neonatal symptoms with minor disabilities at school age. Archives of Disease in Childhood Fetal and Neonatal Edition 86(1):F16–F21

Niklasson A, Albertsson-Wikland K 2008 Continuous growth reference from 24th week of gestation to 24 months by gender. BMC Pediatrics 8(8):1–14

Payne VG, Isaacs LD 2008 Human motor development: a lifespan approach, 7th edn. McGraw-Hill, New York

Ponseti IV, Morcuende JA, Mosca V et al 2003 Clubfoot: Ponseti management, 2nd edn. Global HELP Publication. Online. Available at: http://www.global-help.org/publications/books/book_cfponseti.html (accessed 4 May 2009)

Ponseti IV, Zhivkov M, Davis N et al 2006 Treatment of the complex idiopathic clubfoot. Clinical Orthopaedics and Related Research 451: 171–176

Sarrafian SK 1993 Anatomy of the foot and ankle, 2nd edn. JB Lippincott, Philadelphia

Shepherd RB 1995 Physiotherapy in paediatrics, 3rd edn. Butterworth Heinemann, Oxford

Tachdjian MO 1985 The child's foot. WB Saunders, Philadelphia

Tachdjian MO 1997 Clinical pediatric orthopedics. Appleton & Lange, Stamford, CT

Talamillo A, Bastida M, Fernandez-Teran M 2005 The developing limb and the control of the number of digits. Clinical Genetics 67:143–153

Thomson P 1993 Introduction to podopaediatrics. WB Saunders, London

Further reading

Embryology – Carnegie stages. Online. Available at: http://embryology.med.unsw.edu.au/wwwhuman/Stages/CStages.htm (accessed 3 May 2009)

Sarrafian SK 1993 Anatomy of the foot and ankle, 2nd edn. Lippincott, Philadelphia

Thomson P 2001 Introduction to podopaediatrics, 2nd edn. WB Saunders, London

Basic bones of ontogeny

Introduction

The newborn infant's skeleton consists of largely cartilaginous 'bone' which is altered by external stresses over time. These forces and stresses are encountered in utero and continue, with the addition of direct gravity, postnatally.

One extreme example of the plasticity of the developing human foot is illustrated by the former traditional practice of binding the feet of baby girls in China. It was thought that the smaller the girl's foot, the greater her marriage prospects and the greater the dowry – with no account being taken of how painfully crippled she might be. This process is described in hideous detail in Jung Chang's memoir *Wild Swans* (Chang 1991).

Less distressing and more commonly encountered forces which affect the infant skeleton arise from:

- intrauterine position
- sleeping positions
- sitting postures.

All can cause significant problems in the development and growth of the paediatric lower limb (Fig. 3.1A, B).

Twins and all multiple births are more susceptible to forces which can mould soft tissues and young bones. Hip instability,

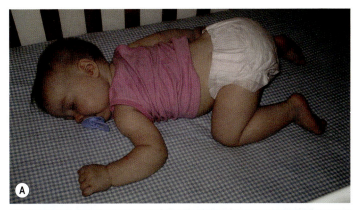

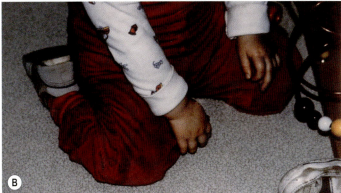

Figure 3.1 (A) Prone posture: birth to 1 month (depicted here in an older infant). Note the overall posture of flexion including: kyphosis of the spine, posterior pelvic tilt, hip and knee flexion. The baby's posture is also one of asymmetrical alignment.
(B) Some intoeing gait is associated with sitting with hips and feet rotated medially.

increased bone shaft torsions and metatarsus adductus have all been related to shared, and hence relatively reduced, intrauterine space (Fig. 3.2).

Historical perspective

In the 1940s, it became clinically evident that the growing skeleton would respond to modelling influences when deformities secondary to poliomyelitis were successfully treated and prevented using braces, splints and

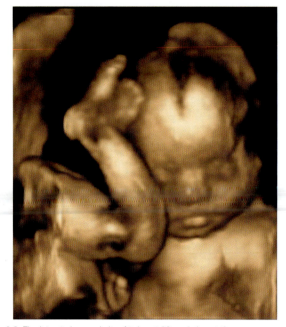

Figure 3.2 The intrauterine proximity of twins at 22 weeks' gestation.

surgical transfers of muscle tendons. With the work of Sabin and Salk, poliomyelitis has been successfully vaccinated against and has dramatically declined in the developed world but it is still seen in children in poorer developing countries. The skills in managing lower limb deformities have now been adopted in the management of cerebral palsy, which, with the advent of amniocentesis and abortion choice, has also declined in prevalence.

Two decades later, in the 1960s, it was found that the abnormal forces produced from spastic muscle contractions caused the deforming of structures being produced from normal bone development. Previously it had been thought that the bony deformities in spastic children were due to abnormal cartilage/bone development. This was quite a step forward in understanding and redirected treatment approaches to be more functional in addition to the use of passive splinting.

Anatomical overview

The lower limb consists skeletally of:

- long bones
- short bones
- sesamoid bones
- accessory bones, if present.

Long bones are tubular (e.g. femur, tibia, fibula, metatarsals, phalanges) while short bones are more cuboidal (e.g. the tarsal bones). Sesamoid bones develop within particular tendons (e.g. patella) and are located at the junction of tendons crossing the ends of long bones (e.g. flexor hallucis brevis and first metatarsal) and function in assisting tendon leverage. Accessory or 'supernumerary' bones develop when extra ossification centres appear and form additional bones (e.g. navicular and os tibiale externum which has approximately 10% incidence).

Heterotopic bones are unusual and form within soft tissues (e.g. scars) as a result of calcification of small muscular haemorrhages (may be referred to as 'rider's bones' when found in the adductors of horse riders; Moore & Dalley 1999).

All skeletal bones are derived from the embryonic mesenchyme either by *direct intramembranous ossification* or by *endochondral ossification*, i.e. via a cartilage template.

There is no difference in histology of bones formed by intramembranous ossification or endochondral ossification. As it is endochondral ossification which largely pertains to the lower limb, a brief outline is included below:

- Mesenchyme differentiates into chondroblasts.
- Chondroblasts form a cartilaginous bone model.
- Cartilaginous bone model calcifies centrally and capillaries infiltrate the interior of the bone model.
- Capillaries and osteogenic cells form a periosteal bud or primary ossification centre.
- Primary ossification centre becomes the diaphysis (Cusick 1990, Moore & Dalley 1999).

Diaphysis

- Comprises the main cortical structure of a long bone.
- The process of endochondral ossification involves progressive destruction and replacement of the hyaline cartilage model.

- Cartilaginous pre-forms precede osseous forms.
- Many eventual skeletal deformities are due to chondrification error, after which normal bony modelling and ossification occur → abnormal skeletal structure.

Metaphyses

- Located at diaphyseal poles.
- Characterized by less cortical thickness and more trabecular bone.
- Prior to completion of mineralization, trabecular bone may be modelled by force.
- Very porous and highly vascular.

Epiphyses

- Secondary ossification centres, located at either end of the diaphysis (the only short bone to develop a secondary ossification centre is the calcaneus; Fig. 3.3).
- Totally cartilaginous at birth with the exception of the distal femur and proximal tibia.
- Epiphyseal arteries infiltrate as do osteogenic cells (e.g. osteoblasts).
- Throughout growth cartilage is progressively replaced by bone, leaving articular cartilage (hyaline) at skeletal maturation.
- Epiphyses with a tendon attached are termed *apophyses* and are predisposed to avulsion injury (e.g. distal fibula, base fifth metatarsal, anterior tibial tubercle).

Physis

- Bony growth plates which intervene between the diaphysis and epiphyses during long bone growth.
- Vulnerable to mechanical disruption, especially from shearing forces.
- Consists of several cellular layers embedded in ground substance.
- Growth ceases when the growth plates are completely replaced by bone fusing the epiphysis with the diaphysis. This usually occurs 1–2 years earlier in girls than boys for the same anatomical sites.
- The resulting synostosis is seen on X-ray as an epiphyseal line which indicates cessation of bone length growth.
- Growth disturbance should always be considered with any physeal injury.

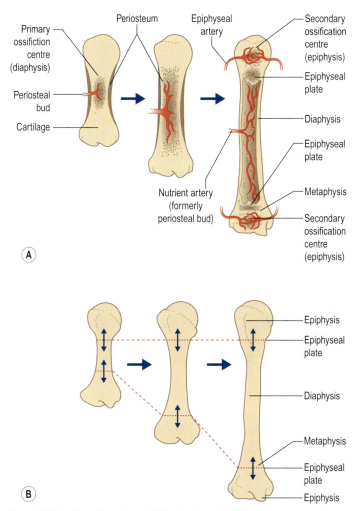

Figure 3.3 Formation of long bones. (A) The development of both primary and secondary ossification centres. (B) The blue arrows indicate that growth occurs on both sides of the cartilaginous epiphyseal growth plates until maturity, when the adjacent sides fuse.

Abridged summary of bone properties

New trabecular bone matrix becomes mineralized after 1 week of formation and mineralization continues for approximately 6 months until complete ossification is achieved. Increased mineralization results in increased bony resilience and reduced strain (deformation due to force) when loads are applied.

Key Concepts

> Younger bone will strain (deform, bend) more than older, more mineralized bone which is why the incomplete cortical or greenstick fracture may be seen in children but not in fully ossified adults.

Bone generally remodels in response to normal physiological stresses.

Muscle activity and joint motion result in forces which strain and influence eventual bony modelling (also the preceding chondral changes) and eventual morphology. Body weight resulting in stress loading is less influential than strain loads on bony formation (Brukner & Khan 1993). Muscular forces provide the major loads, with the nervous system contributing to chondral modelling via muscle innervation control (hence children with increased tonicity have increased neuron-motor forces associated with bone development).

Overall skeletal formation is not just due to primary or isolated bone growth. The fetal osseous 'blueprint' is influenced by postnatal skeletal use but primarily determined by genetic factors.

A physical law of bony adaptation (attributed to Wolff) states that bone is deposited in areas subjected to stress/strain and resorbed from areas of minimal forces, i.e. 'form follows function'. Bony modelling occurs due to simultaneous osteoblastic deposition and opposing osteoclastic resorption, e.g. resolution of developmental genu varum/valgum.

Growth, by definition, occurs when bone deposition exceeds bone resorption.

Fractures

Bone fractures occur when bones are loaded beyond their yield point (Thomson 1993). Fractures are quite common in children and usually heal quite rapidly as a result of the potent remodelling ability of young bone (Fig. 3.4). Fractures in children occur more often than ligament injuries or dislocations due to the strength of bone versus ligaments. This changes with increasing age, such that more ligament injuries and joint dislocations are seen in older people.

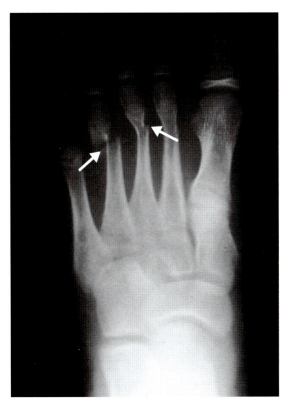

Figure 3.4 Metatarsal shaft fractures in a child aged 8 years.

There is a classification system for fractures which is fairly universal and helps to organize management planning (Slongo & Audige 2008). Usually fractures are classified according to their cause and type.

Causes

i. *Trauma*: due to a single episode of a large, externally applied force.

ii. *Stress*: results from repeated loads applied to the one site which eventually cause the bone to fatigue.

iii. *Pathology*: due to systemically abnormal bones or a discrete lesion such as a bone cyst which creates a weakened site more likely to yield to forced loading.

Types (Fig. 3.5)

i. Transverse:
- a one-plane fracture perpendicular to the shaft of a long bone
- usually stable once reduced.

ii. Oblique:
- a one-plane fracture which runs obliquely across the shaft
- the bone may shorten if the fracture slides.

iii. Spiral:
- can appear similar to an oblique fracture if viewed in just one plane, but actually curves obliquely across all three planes of the bone shaft
- prone to shortening by rotation.

iv. Comminuted:
- results in fragmentation of bone within the long bone shaft
- lacks stability.

v. Crush:
- occurs in bones which are largely cancellous (spongy) in form rather than those with outer cortical bone strength, as in types i–iv.
- the calcaneus and the vertebrae are prone to crush fractures.

vi. Avulsion:
- seen especially in children, the avulsion fracture sees a piece of bone torn away by its tendon or ligament attachment (Brukner & Khan 1993). The same injury mechanism in older people sees damage to the tendon or ligament rather than the young, softer bone (e.g. ankle inversion sprain which commonly sees rupture of the ATFL in adults but in a child may avulse the distal fibula).

In addition a fracture may be:

Open or closed:	bone exposed or not.
Complicated:	nerve or blood vessel damage, infection, mal-union.
Greenstick or buckle:	these only occur in children as the young, less mineralized and hence less brittle bones can bend without fully breaking. Greenstick fractures are incomplete fractures on the bent side of the bone. Buckle fractures occur with cortical compression along the metaphysis as commonly occurs after a fall on an outstretched arm.

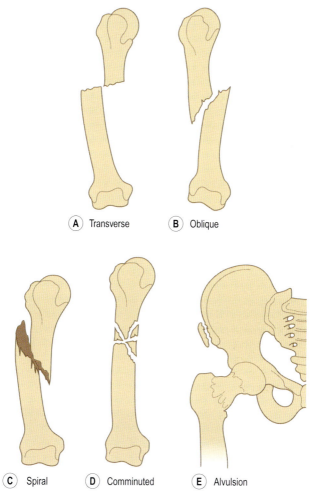

Figure 3.5 Fracture classification diagrams. The avulsion fracture is seen particularly in children, and occurs when bone attached to ligament or tendon is torn from the main body.

The remodelling capacity of bone is dependent upon the:

- age of the child
- distance of injury from the end of the bone
- angulation.

As a principle, remodelling will occur if:

- more than 2 years of bone growth remains
- fracture is near the dynamic area of the epiphyseal plate
- deformity is in the plane of associated motion.

Remodelling will not occur with:

- displaced intra-articular fracture
- diaphyseal fractures which are shortened or rotated (usually from types ii–iv)
- displaced fractures perpendicular to the plane of motion
- displaced fractures crossing the growth plate at 90°.

A separate classification system exists for growth plate or epiphyseal fractures (Fig. 3.6). The Salter–Harris classification deals with acute fractures of a growth plate and injuries are classified as follows:

Types I and II – horizontal fractures.
Types III and IV – vertical fractures.
Type V – compression fracture.

Types I and II represent a lower risk to bone growth disruption than types III and IV, which involve the joint surface. Types III and IV nearly always require ORIF (open reduction with internal fixation) (Schnetzler & Hoernschemeyer 2007). Type V is rare and is usually only diagnosed retrospectively once growth disturbance is noted (Bloomfield et al 1992).

Muscles

As muscle leverage influences both fractures and joints, it is suitable to briefly discuss skeletal muscle at this juncture.

By way of review, there are three basic types of muscles:

1. skeletal
2. cardiac
3. smooth.

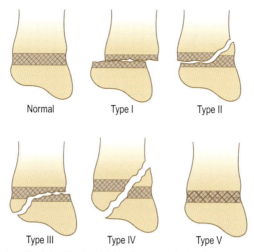

Figure 3.6 A modified classification of Salter–Harris growth plate fractures. Types III and IV involve the articular surfaces and usually require surgical reduction and fixation. Growth disturbance may ensue.

While the musculature of the heart (cardiac) and blood vessels and organs (smooth) are vitally important, it is skeletal muscle which is more pertinent for podiatrists as it is intrinsic to movement and gait. Skeletal muscles are attached to bones (or cartilage, fascia, ligaments) via tendons. The proximal attachment or *origin* is usually stable while the distal attachment or *insertion* is the movable part during muscle contraction (this is generally the case, but not exclusively so).

As the name suggests, a musculo-tendinous unit comprises both the muscle belly and its tendinous attachments at either end. The muscle bellies in the lower limb are generally fleshy with long muscle fibres running in parallel bundles. The muscle fibres are made up of smaller myofibrils. Movement per se is derived from activation of the *motor unit*, the coupling of a motor neuron and muscle fibre (Moore & Dalley 1999) (Fig. 3.7).

Motion results from activation of many motor units (Moore & Dalley 1999). Muscles function during body movements as:

Agonists: main drivers of a specific motion.
Antagonists: oppose the agonist to create a smooth movement.

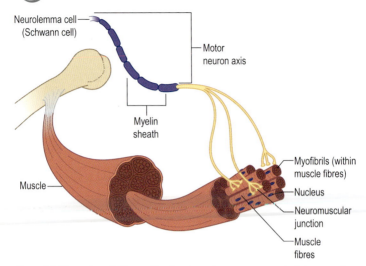

Figure 3.7 The motor unit. The combination of a motor neuron axon and all-sized muscle fibres constitutes a motor unit.

Synergists: complement the agonist by preventing movement at any intervening joints spanned by the agonist.

Fixators: function to stabilize a proximal part of the limb while motion occurs more distally.

Joints

Joints have varying functions and are generally classified as one of three types:

- synovial
- fibrous
- cartilaginous.

Synovial joints

Synovial joints include articular cartilage on adjacent bone ends which are housed within an articular capsule containing synovial fluid. These are the most common type of joint and typify the limb joints.

Features of synovial joints include:

- Articular cartilage on apposing ends of bones.
- Joint cavity (lined with synovial membrane).
- An enclosing articular capsule.

Synovial joints have free movements between the bones involved and are stabilized by surrounding and/or intrinsic ligaments. Some synovial joints also have fibrocartilaginous discs interposing the bony surfaces, e.g. between the spinal vertebrae.

Synovial joints are further sub-classified depending upon shape or joint movement:

i. Plane – e.g. gliding.

ii. Hinge – one-plane range, i.e. flexion, extension.

iii. Saddle – two-plane range, i.e. surfaces are concave against convex.

iv. Condyloid – two-plane range with one plane dominating.

v. Ball and socket – three-plane range, i.e. high ranges of motion, e.g. hip joint.

vi. Pivot – one-plane joint which allows rotation only, e.g. atlas-axis (C2 vertebrae).

Fibrous joints

Fibrous joints are joined by fibrous tissue to form syndesmoses composed of either ligament or fibrous membrane. The skull sutures are examples of fibrous joints.

Cartilaginous joints

Cartilaginous joints are joined by either fibrocartilage or hyaline cartilage to form synchondroses. The epiphyseal growth plates are examples of primary (or temporary) cartilaginous joints involving hyaline cartilage. Secondary cartilaginous joints, such as those joining the intervertebral discs, involve fibrocartilage which provides strength, shock attenuation and flexibility.

The effects of exercise

We know that exercise increases bone mineral density (BMD) and that a consistent lack of exercise is associated with reduced BMD (Payne & Isaacs 2008). Children who are chronically ill and bed-or chair-bound will exhibit considerable loss of BMD. Studies suggest that low physical activity is a risk factor for reduced lumbar bone mass in children with haemophilia (Larson & Henderson 2000, Tlacuilo-Parra et al 2008). This factor must be monitored to avoid reduction in BMD that might contribute to further skeletal fragility. Calcium supplements are ineffective in the absence of exercise (Ward et al 2007).

Key *Concepts*

Cross-training is advisable for young sports participants for many reasons. BMD will be optimized in children who are involved in a variety of sports and activities and skills are enhanced more comprehensively than when a single sport occurs (Gibson et al 2004).

Particular regard is due for the young female athlete in terms of relationship between BMD and exercise (Fenichel & Warren 2007). The so-called female athlete triad occurs when girls try to reduce too much body fat (unfortunately some develop eating disorders in the process), amenorrhoea occurs (absence of menstruation) and subsequently osteoporosis as BMD falls (Benjamin 2007).

References

Benjamin HJ 2007 The female adolescent athlete: specific concerns. Pediatric Annals 36(11):719–726

Bloomfield J, Fricker PA, Fitch KD 1992 Textbook of science and medicine in sport. Blackwell Scientific Publications, Melbourne

Brukner P, Khan K 1993 Clinical sports medicine. McGraw-Hill, Sydney

Chang J 1991 Wild swans: three daughters in China. Flamingo, Harper Collins, London

Cusick BD 1990 Progressive casting and splinting for lower extremity deformities in children with neuromotor dysfunction. Therapy Skill Builders, Arizona

Fenichel RM, Warren MP 2007 Anorexia, bulimia, and the athletic triad: evaluation and management. Current Osteoporosis Reports 5(4):160–164

Gibson JH, Mitchell A, Harries MG 2004 Nutritional and exercise-related determinants of bone density in elite female runners. Osteoporosis International 15(8):611–618

Larson CM, Henderson RC 2000 Bone mineral density and fractures in boys with Duchenne muscular dystrophy. Journal of Pediatric Orthopedics 20(1):71–74

Moore KL, Dalley AF 1999 Clinically orientated anatomy, 4th edn. Lipincott, Williams and Wilkins, Baltimore

Payne VG, Isaacs LD 2008 Human motor development: a lifespan approach, 7th edn. McGraw-Hill, New York

Schnetzler KA, Hoernschemeyer D 2007 The pediatric triplane ankle fracture. Journal of the American Academy of Orthopaedic Surgeons 15(12):738–747

Slongo TF, Audige L 2008 Fracture and dislocation classification compendium for children: the AO pediatric comprehensive classification of long bone fractures (PCCF). Journal of Orthopaedic Trauma 21(10 Suppl.):S135–S160

Thomson P 1993 Introduction to podopaediatrics. WB Saunders, London

Tlacuilo-Parra A, Morales-Zambrano R, Lopez-Guido B et al 2008 Inactivity is a risk factor for low bone mineral density among haemophilic children. British Journal of Haematology 140(5):562–567

Ward KA, Roberts SA, Adams JE 2007 Calcium supplementation and weight bearing physical activity – do they have a combined effect on the bone density of pre-pubertal children? Bone 41(4):496–504

Further reading

Moore KL, Dalley AF 1999 Clinically orientated anatomy. Lippincott, Williams and Wilkins, Baltimore

Sarrafian SK 1993 Anatomy of the foot and ankle. JB Lippincott, Philadelphia

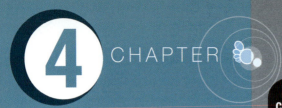

Developmental biomechanics

Definition of developmental biomechanics

The study of the effects of externally applied forces on the musculoskeletal system during early life.

Introduction

This chapter does not provide the reader with an exhaustive account but rather attempts to provide an overview of the gross morphological development of the lower limb and foot from birth to maturity, so that these notable aspects of development of the lower limb and foot can be appreciated in such a way that useful clinical benchmarks ensue.

Clearly, it is only by understanding the normal development of the lower limb that clinical abnormalities can be distinguished from developmentally expected parameters. A classic example of the importance of this distinction occurs at the knee, where genu varum is clinically normal in an infant aged 6 months, yet clinically abnormal in a child aged 4 years. Knowledge of developmental traits and variants are essential for the clinician in both the detection of problems and an appreciation of normal physiologic growth. Tempering the need for clinical benchmarks is the appreciation that a wide spectrum of 'normal' is encountered.

Spine

The newborn spine is kyphotic, with the vertebral column from cervical to sacral level being a continuous flexion curve (as viewed laterally). The proportions of the segments of the spine are vastly different to those of the adult, with the cervical and lumbar lengths approximating some 25% each of the total length.

Imaging the young spine

Spinal sonography can be performed in newborns and young infants as long as the vertebral arches are not completely ossified. Indications for spinal sonography are midline cutaneous markers in the lumbosacral region, subcutaneous masses, foot abnormalities, anorectal and genitourinary malformations and neurological abnormalities of the lower extremities. All these clinical symptoms are suspicious of spina bifida occulta and tethered cord which should be ruled out by spinal sonography (Deeg et al 2007).

Sonography of the neonatal spine is now accepted as a highly sensitive, readily available screening study that can be used to evaluate various anomalies of the lumbar spine in most infants younger than 4 months (Lowe et al 2007). Fetal magnetic resonance imaging (MRI) is an increasingly available technique used to evaluate the fetal brain and spine. This is made possible by recent advances in technology and it affords a unique opportunity for studying in vivo brain development and early diagnosis of congenital abnormalities inadequately visualized or undetectable by prenatal sonography (Glenn & Barkovich 2006).

Working against gravity

Development of the neuromuscular system results in many antigravity motions of the infant which has the net effect of mobilizing the spine from flexion to extension. These movements should be occurring and actively observable by 6 months of age (Fig. 4.1).

Key Concepts

It is important to appreciate the concept that modelling of bony structures is a dynamic process. Fed by the maturation of the neurological system, muscle activity and resulting movements direct forces across young bones and joints to direct eventual morphological form (Guidera et al 1994).

Students might like to remember the following motto:
'It's the nerves, which drive the muscles, to shape the bones.'

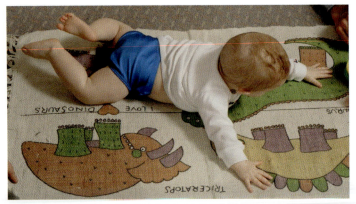

Figure 4.1 A 6-month-old child showing typical antigravity floor skills.

Typical movements and ages at which these emerge are:

- Head lift: 2 months (asymmetrical).
- 'Frog leg' and kick: 3 months.
- 'Swimming':   4–5 months.
- Tummy crawl: 6 months.
- Quadruped rock: 7 months.

It is important for the prone and supine skills to be balanced, which has important implications for positioning the infant.

Sudden infant death syndrome (SIDS)

Parents in the 1950s were very influenced by the manual for babies and infants written by Dr Benjamin Spock. Parents were advised to lie babies prone for sleeping, a practice which was later identified as being associated with SIDS and is now warned against. The practice of lying babies supine has altered motor development by delaying the attainment of skills gained from prone positioning. Plagiocephaly is also more common and children's health clinics now advocate regular 'tummy time' when babies are awake to build strength from prone posture. The risk for sudden infant death syndrome in black infants is twice that of white infants, and their parents are twice as likely to place them in the prone position for sleep (Colson et al 2006, Moon et al 2004).

On their feet

The newly standing and, in many cases, walking 1-year-old child displays an anterior pelvic tilt. Adjustment of the pelvic tilt allows for centre of gravity adaptation with growth, ranging from 18 to 40° (iliac crest angulation to transverse plane).

The typical 'pot belly' appearance of the 2-year-old child occurs due to lumbar hyperextension in combination with anterior pelvic tilt. This continues to form a structural lumbar lordosis which counterbalances with developmental genu recurvatum in the 2–3-year-old child.

Lordotic curvature in the lumbar region increases during ages 4–7 years, reaching the maximal value of approximately 30–40° anterior pelvic tilt by 7 years. Tightness of structures such as the hamstrings may result in a greater than usual anterior pelvic tilt or may see the degree of pelvic tilt reached at an earlier age. This is more marked in children with muscular hypertonicity (Fig. 4.2). Referral to either a physiotherapist

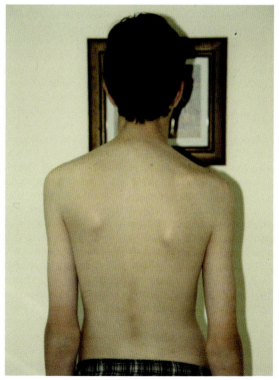

Figure 4.2 Unilateral hamstring tightness may be associated with scoliosis, evidenced by the scapular heights.

or an orthopaedist for more comprehensive assessment may be indicated, and is also indicated with observation of other asymmetry, such as one very pronated foot versus a normal foot (functional limb length discrepancy). Subtle asymmetry does not necessarily require intervention.

Pelvic tilt and lumbar lordosis, two position-dependent factors, increase with age, to avoid inadequate anterior displacement of the body centre of gravity (Mac-Thiong et al 2004).

Pelvis

The newborn pelvis is small and tilted posteriorly in the sagittal plane, even more so when the infant is positioned prone.

The acetabular cup is shallow and faces inferiorly in the sagittal plane. By 3 years of age the acetabular cup angles further inferiorly.

The hip joint is in a position of flexion and lateral rotation due to the combined forces of surrounding ligaments and muscles. Both capsular ligament contracture and also contracture of hip flexors and lateral rotator muscles are involved in this posture. There are twice as many lateral rotators as medial rotators at the hip joint.

The posture of the newborn baby reflects the 'close packed' position in utero in the last trimester of pregnancy (Fig. 4.3). Note the flexion/abduction of hips, knee flexion, medial tibial position, ankle dorsiflexion, relative adduction of the feet. The stress of this close packed positioning stabilizes joint complexes. The rapidly increasing size of the fetus from 22 to 24 weeks' gestation means that the available space for the developing body becomes diminished, necessitating the closely wrapped position of flexion of most joints. Thus, post-birth, the direction of musculoskeletal development is one which reduces this flexed and tightly packed posture to one which in approximately 10–16 months sees the child extended and bipedal.

Around the hip joints we see the necessary reduction of flexion and lateral rotation (the infant is no longer physically confined) due to the activation of muscle groups and the simultaneous stretching of ligaments. Together these forces shape the osseous structures. The following brief and very simplified description in relation to the hip may assist in understanding the basic concepts of this bony modelling process:

- the acetabular cup deepens and angles more inferiorly
- due to the force of placement of the head of femur
- which is moved 'into' the acetabulum

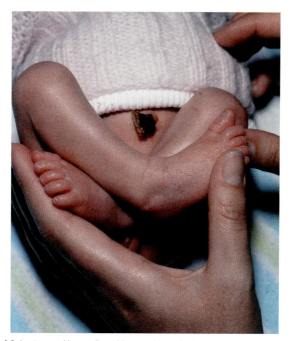

Figure 4.3 In utero position, replicated in a newborn infant.

- with reduced hip joint flexion and lateral rotation
- following the end of intrauterine confinement, activation of hip extensors, elongation of anterior pelvic capsular ligaments.

The aim of this process is to produce a stable hip joint for eventual bipedal weight-bearing. It is important to remember that the maturation of the nervous system sees activity occurring in the muscles, which through their agonist–antagonist pairing, place modelling forces through young plastic bones and ligaments, resulting in the eventual skeletal form. Postures in the infant may also be influential to a lesser degree on eventual skeletal form and often have cultural association (e.g. swaddling with legs extended versus carrying on backs with abducted, flexed hips).

Developmental dysplasia of the hip (DDH)

Early detection, diagnosis and treatment of developmental dysplasia of the hip (DDH; previously known as congenital hip dislocation) are essential in preventing further disability and reduced quality of life for affected children. In a study of 8145 infants, the rate of suspected DDH was 0.95% and that of diagnosed DDH was 0.63% (Stein-Zamir et al 2008). Children with DDH have the following demographic and perinatal risk markers:

- female
- first born
- breech presentation
- oligohydramnios.

Key Concepts

The highest positive predictive value (95.5%) in physical evaluation was any sign of a dislocatable hip, as assessed using Ortolani's or Barlow's tests (Shepherd 1995). DDH diagnosis after 6 weeks of age was associated with a higher likelihood of surgery and motor disability.

Clinical screening to enable early diagnosis of DDH is essential to avoid later problems (Fig. 4.4).

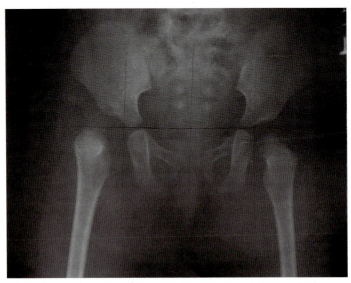

Figure 4.4 Developmental hip dysplasia (left). This child, detected at 2.5 years of age, was walking with a noticeable limp and 'short' left leg appearance.

Hip joint range of motion

Hip joint range of motion is in three cardinal body planes:

1. Sagittal

At birth the hip is flexed some 30°. The iliofemoral and ischiofemoral ligaments together with the iliopsoas muscle are short and inactive and aid in this position of flexion. Gluteus maximus and the proximal portion of adductor magnus become active and antagonize these structures with their function as hip extensors.

The clinical test for hip extension range is Staheli's prone hip extension test. From 3 years the normal hip extension is 0°, which in part accounts for the short stride length in children under 3 years (adults usually have 55° of hip extension/flexion).

Hip flexion contracture of 15–20° is an indication for surgical lengthening as approximately 15° of hip extension is required for the child to walk normally. Hip extension is an abnormal finding in gestation.

2. Transverse

Until age 2 years, the range of lateral rotation in the transverse plane at the hip joint exceeds that of medial rotation. Coupled with this change in proportion of motion is reduction in the quantity of motion, from 120–150° in the newborn to approximately 100° by age 2 years. Anteversion reduces simultaneously with antetorsion (defined below, under Femur), but involves different structures.

3. Frontal/coronal

The hip joint is abducted 75° in the neonate (while flexed) and this is reduced to 60° by approximately 9 months of age. In the 2-year-old child the normal amount of hip abduction is 45°, which remains fairly static into adulthood.

Coxa valga (angle between the head/neck axis and the femoral shaft axis in the frontal plane) measures up to 150° in the neonate, reducing to its mature value of 125–135° by 6 years.

Femur

The femur is the largest bone in the body and its development is almost as contentious and confusing in terms of nomenclature.

The terms anteversion and antetorsion (and counterparts, retroversion and retrotorsion) are used with variation by many authors due to divergence of definition (Fabry et al 1994, Valmassy 1996). For the purpose of clarity we adopt the definitions of Cusick (Cusick 1990, Cusick & Stuberg 1992):

Torsion (femoral):

'A medial twist in the shaft of the bone, distal on proximal.'

Version (femoral):

'A positional change in which either the acetabulum or the head and neck of the femur are directed anteriorly, relative to the frontal plane. The head and neck of the femur are maintained in this alignment by soft tissue, including ligament, muscle, and joint capsule.'

There are three distinct growth plates in the proximal femur which contribute to growth:

- Longitudinal growth plate: contributes 30% to femur length.
- Trochanteric growth plate: contributes to modelling of femoral head and neck.
- Femoral neck isthmus.

The proximal femur is composed entirely of hyaline cartilage in the neonate and is thus very pliable in infancy and early childhood.

The newborn femur shows:

- coxa valga
- femoral torsion (medial)
- mild varus bowing
- some anterior bowing.

Each of these femoral attributes indicates skeletal immaturity due to intrauterine position and fetal skeletal design.

Coxa valga

Describes the angle formed between the femoral neck and shaft.

Approximates 150° in the neonate and reduces with age to 125–135° at 6 years, 125° in the adult.

Table 4.1 provides a summary of the most commonly assessed aspects of the lower limb (excluding the foot) and normative values across main research studies (Beeson 1999, Cheng et al 1991, Cusick & Stuberg 1992, Eckhoff & Johnson 1994, Fabry et al 1994, Guidera et al 1994, Heath & Staheli 1993, Jacquemier et al 2008, Kumar & MacEwen 1982, Pasciak et al 1996, Schneider et al 1997, Staheli 1989).

Table 4.1 Compilation of values for main attributes of lower limb profile development (across multiple studies)

	Hip	Femur	Knee	Tibia	Thigh–foot
Age (years)	**Position**	**Torsion**	**Position**	**Torsion**	**Angle**
0–2	Medial hip range: 43° age 2 years Lateral hip range: 40° at 2 years	Average: Females: >40° medial at birth Males: 30°	Genu varum at birth averages 10°, abnormal after 2 years	Minimal at birth	Average: −10° to 0° (range −25° to 20°)
3–4		Average Females: 40° medial (SD 20°) Males: 28° (18°)	Genu valgum: maximizes with 8–12° valgus at 3–4 years	TMA averages 34° lateral (SD 6°)	15° abducted after age 2–3 years
7–8		Average Females: 28° medial (SD 20°) Males: 14° (14°)	Genu valgum: reduces to <5°	*Torsion averages 20° lateral (range 0–45°) by ages 7–8 years	
9–12	Medial hip range: 56° by 9 years Lateral hip range: 30° at 9 years	Average Females: 10–15° medial by age 10 years (SD 15°) Males: 10° (14°)	Genu valgum > 10° is abnormal	*TMA averages 35° lateral (SD 4°)	Averages 10° abducted (range −5° to 35°) at age 12 years
Adult	45° medial 45° lateral	15° medial (females) 5° medial (males)		Torsion 20° TMA 35°	10° abducted

*Method of assessment: CT values (torsion) approx. 10° less than TMA method.

Femoral torsion

Describes the medial twist in the shaft of the bone, distal on proximal end.
At birth there is approximately 40° of medial femoral torsion.
By 2 years 30° of femoral torsion remains, having reduced due to:

- Reduced hip flexion contracture.
- Activation of hip extensors and lateral rotators (which put a torsional modelling force through the proximal third of the cartilaginous femur).

Key Concepts

Reduction of femoral torsion is greatest in the first 2 years (from approximately 40° to 30°) and again at puberty (from approximately 25° to 15°).

The adult femoral torsion range varies according to different studies (and individuals): 5–15° (Cusick 1990).

The mean value of femoral torsion measured using ultrasound in 97 children aged 6 and 15 years was 37° in the 6-year-old group and 24° in the 15-year-old group. The mean value of tibial torsion was 18° in both age groups. Neither side- nor sex-dependent differences in both age groups were found (Pasciak et al 1996).

Average femoral torsion measured using magnetic resonance imaging (MRI) was 10.4°. MRI provides an alternative to computed tomography (CT) in the measurement of femoral and tibial torsion (Schneider et al 1997).

Key Concepts

Clinical assessment of torsion of the femur is estimated using Ryder's test. This clinical test indirectly assesses the torsional status of the femur and has been found to demonstrate good reliability and validity in the hands of experienced examiners. It may, however, underestimate femoral torsion in some children with cerebral palsy due to altered trochanteric sites (Cusick 1990, Cusick & Stuberg 1992, Davids et al 2002; Figs 4.5, 4.6).

Knee

Similarly to the hip joint, the newborn's knee exhibits flexion contracture as a normal finding. Accompanying this position are the attitudes of genu varum and medial genicular position.

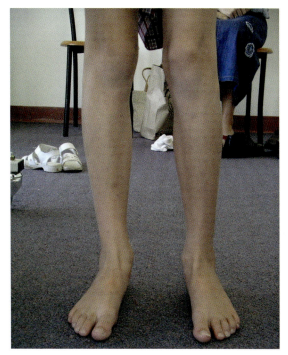

Figure 4.5 Femoral torsion. A 12-year-old girl with residual increased medial femoral torsion (**R > L**) as shown by her patellae positioning and which was measurable using Ryder's test clinically.

Knee joint in three cardinal body planes

1. Sagittal plane

The knee of the neonate is flexed approximately 30° due to:

a. intrauterine positioning → adaptive shortening of soft tissues
b. maturation of the nervous system → flexor muscle activity.

These two factors combine to result in 'physiologic flexion' in newborns as observed in elbows, hips, ankles and knees.

Normal development sees reduction of this flexion by 6 months of age, assisted by the infant's 'mouthing' of their feet, an activity which actively assists in elongating hamstrings both actively and passively. Infants continue to elongate their hamstrings and hence reduce knee

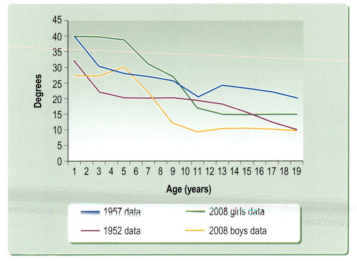

Figure 4.6 This summary of two studies from the 1950s (both had over 200 subjects) identified the same trend in reducing femoral torsion with increasing age, but values varied due to hip positioning and examiner technique (Cusick 1990). The 2008 data (over 1300 children) separate girls and boys and show appreciable gender difference with greater femoral torsion as a part of the female profile (Jacquemier et al 2008).

flexion, by standing and later moving to begin the bear stand/walk posture.

2. Transverse plane

Flexion of the knee allows medial rotation of the tibia on the distal femur. Intrauterine confinement flexes the knee, rotating the tibiofibular unit medial to result in the medial genicular position on the newborn lower legs. There are more muscles crossing the knee medially than laterally such that flexion denotes medial rotation. There is also adaptive tightness of ligaments and joint capsule from intrauterine positioning.

The ligaments and joint capsule must stretch to allow lateral rotation of the tibiofibular unit on the distal femur as occurs with knee extension. This lateral rotation is essential for knee stability and efficient 'locking' and 'unlocking' functioning in later gait. The initial medial genicular position needs to reduce to allow for adequate lateral rotation with knee extension.

Approximately 5° of lateral rotation of the tibiofibular unit occurs in the last 10° of knee extension to make the knee congruent. Increased transverse plane range of motion in children under 3 years reflects the connective tissue and muscular mobility of this osseous unstable joint.

Medial genicular bias If lateral rotation capacity is less than or not greater than 0° on the transverse plane of the knee joint, such that a medially rotated position of the tibiofibular unit is not reducible and persists, the knee is described as having a *medial genicular bias*. In contrast to the normally occurring medial genicular position, a medial genicular bias deprives the knee joint of any lateral rotation range of motion and may require intervention (Fig. 4.7).

Medial genicular bias may persist in infants/children with neuromotor dysfunction.

Key *Concepts*

Medial genicular bias is a positional deformity that occurs in the transverse plane within the knee joint and as such must be distinguished from true (and less common) medial tibial torsion, which is an osseous deformity with, to the uninitiated clinician, a similar presentation.

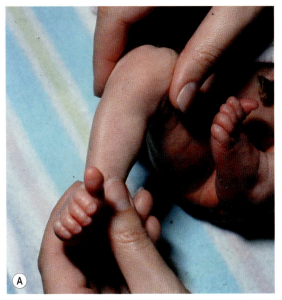

Ⓐ

Figure 4.7 (A) Genicular range: medial range normally predominates (up to age 2 years). Lateral genicular range of motion in this newborn is 0–10°, as shown by the abduction of the foot.

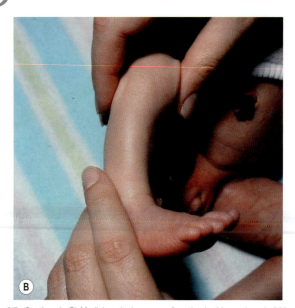

Figure 4.7 *Continued.* (B) Medial genicular range of motion in this newborn is 50°, as shown by the adduction of the foot.

Normal development Usually the infant begins to crawl between the ages of 5 and 9 months. The infant's mobility results in knee extension and accompanying lateral rotation as the infant uses their feet to push and propel their trunk along the floor. This action assists in the reduction of the medial genicular position.

While there is a considerable variation of normal walking ages (10–16 months), most children begin to walk between 12 and 14 months of age as the action of hip and knee extension also promotes lateral rotation of the tibiofibular unit at the knee level.

3. Frontal/coronal plane

The newborn knee exhibits genu varum in the frontal plane, which reduces in the first 6 months and continues to reduce over the first 2 years of life. The degree of varus angulation is disputed between authors with a tibio-femoral angle of up to 17° stated as normal in the newborn (Beeson 1999). Clinically, bowing of the knees is represented by the distance between the medial knee condyles, with opposed tibial malleoli. On average, this distance has been observed as 3 cm in newborns. Normally, there is rapid reduction of genu varum in the first 12–24 months. The intercondylar gap reaches zero by 12–18 months (Cheng et al 1991, Heath & Staheli 1993) and then becomes negative, approximating 3 cm at age 3 years (Cheng et al 1991). Clinically this is now seen as a 3 cm gap at the medial tibial malleoli.

Constituents of developmental genu varum include the following factors:

- coxa valga
- lateral hip rotation (anteversion)
- mild lateral femoral bowing
- medial knee flexion contracture
- medial genicular position.

Normal development sees genu varum resolving by 2 years of age, at which stage the knee is usually straight on the frontal plane (Fig. 4.8). Genu varum after age 2 years is abnormal (Heath & Staheli 1993). Blount's disease is an important diagnostic consideration if genu varum is not reduced or is asymmetrical in children aged 2 years or more (Accadbled et al 2003). Modelling forces on the medial aspect of the knee continue to promote growth and hence the knee progresses into genu valgum, which peaks at approximately 3–4 years with a tibiofemoral angle of 12°. Genu valgum reduces to approximately 5°, which is its mature value (Heath & Staheli 1993). This is usually seen by 8–10 years.

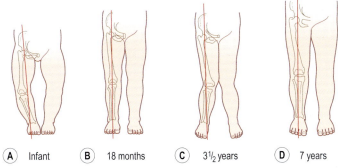

| (A) Infant | (B) 18 months | (C) 3½ years | (D) 7 years |

Figure 4.8 Genu varum to valgum. The normal physiologic transitions, with respect to age, on the frontal/coronal plane.

Modelling forces and the resolution of genu varum, genu valgum

Genu varum and valgum modelling occurs due to variable compressions of the medial and lateral femoral condyles against the tibial condyles in both stance and gait. These compressive forces combine with:

- reduced coxa valga
- reduced medial genicular position
- medial shift of body weight
- reduced foot pronation

to result in the observed increase and decrease in frontal plane angulations at the knee joint with osseous development and growth between birth and 8 years (with possible increase in genu valgum seen at puberty which resolves to the adult genu valgum approximating 5°; Beeson 1999, Heath & Staheli 1993).

The newborn infant exhibits genu varum, which reduces due to less physical confinement and associated hip joint alignments. Figure 4.8 indicates the normal age for frontal plane alignments of the lower limb.

A conceptual approach to bone modelling

Normal compressive forces between bones induce cartilaginous growth and eventual endochondral ossification. For example, in genu varum this position results in a greater compressive force across the medial condyles than across the lateral condyles. As a result, there is an increased rate of medial condylar growth when compared to lateral condylar growth, which resolves the varus angulation.

The continued increased rate of medial condylar growth results in genu valgum, a position which results in greater compressive force across lateral condyles than across medial condyles. In turn, there is an increased rate of lateral condylar growth when compared to medial condylar growth, which assists in resolution of maximum valgus angulation (see Fig. 4.8).

These forces equalize at approximately 5° of genu valgum at the time of proximal tibial physeal closure.

Clinical tests for knee range and position

As stated earlier, it is useful and thorough to examine a joint from the perspective of all three cardinal body planes and to relate this to stance and gait.

1. Sagittal plane

Popliteal angle – test for knee joint extension (Fig. 4.9).

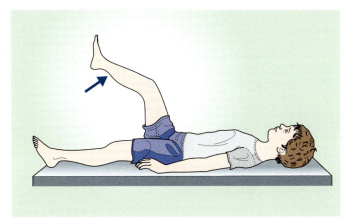

Figure 4.9 Popliteal angle examination.

This test assesses:

- hamstrings
- gastrocnemius
- neural tension (straight leg raise)
- joint capsule
- ligaments.

Basic technique Extend the knee – reduced popliteal angle indicates tight hamstrings. Tight hamstrings are a frequent component of anterior knee pain in sporting youngsters (and adults) and may be a component of the quadriceps group muscle imbalance in Osgood–Schlatter disease.

Dorsiflex the ankle – if popliteal angle reduces further, this indicates tight proximal gastrocnemius.

Extend the hip – if knee remains flexed, this indicates capsular tightness. Rotating the hip medially/laterally will help to discriminate biceps femoris from semimembranosus and semitendinosus.

Be careful to consider neural tension when using this test, as segmental tightening can elicit painful signs (Shacklock 2005).

2. Transverse plane

Genicular rotations – test for genicular ranges, position and detection of joint range bias.

Basic technique Flex the knee and rotate the tibiofibular unit medially and laterally, noting range of motion (Fig. 4.7 A, B).

Greater medial range is often a normal finding in children up 2–3 years, but lateral motion should be available, or the joint is said to be 'biased'.

Test knee rotation ranges with the hip extended and then flexed. If a greater medial range is found in both positions, this indicates tight ligaments. If the medial range changes with the hip position, this indicates tight musculature as well.

The range of motion available in the transverse plane at the knee reduces after 3 years of age, at which time genicular ranges should be even medially and laterally.

Lower leg

The lower leg of the newborn and young child is confusing to examine, as it is difficult to clinically separate the tibia and fibula. In essence, the lower leg at birth exhibits:

- declination of the proximal tibial plateau
- minimal true tibial torsion
- apparent tibial varum (with genu varum)
- a short fibula (Fig. 4.10).

1. Sagittal

The newborn tibial plateau on the transverse plane declines some 25° inferiorly in the sagittal plane.

This is masked by the normal physiologic flexion of the knees and associated with developmental genu recurvatum, which acts as a counterbalance mechanism in the sagittal plane as a lumbar lordosis and the associated anterior tilting of the pelvis occur in the young child. Declination of the tibial plateau reduces to 5° by adolescence.

2. Transverse

In the newborn, the tibia and fibula are quite straight on the transverse plane with minimal end-on-end torsion within the bone shafts, although this can be easily confused on examination. Tibiofibular torsion is difficult to assess clinically, but Lang's research guides the clinician, advocating the following approach (Lang & Volpe 1998):

- proximal tibial condyles are placed in the frontal plane
- transmalleolar axis deviation from the frontal plane is used as an indicator of torsional status.

True tibial torsion is best assessed by CT or MRI, although results are still inconsistent and depend on positioning and technique. Tibial torsion develops laterally, averaging 20° (range 0–45°) by 6–8 years (Fabry et al

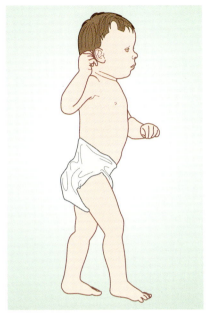

Figure 4.10 Lateral view of new walker, aged 13 months. Factors to note are: residual flexion of all limbs, 'high guard' arm position, lumbar lordosis, leg and trunk length approximate, short stride, absent heel strike, flat, fat medial foot arch area.

1994). This occurs due to crawling, walking and standing tiptoe, all of which apply a lateral torque across the tibia and fibula. The distal tibia and fibula are almost entirely cartilaginous and hence very pliable and responsive to applied torques.

3. Frontal

The legs of the newborn have long been observed to appear bowed on the frontal plane. In fact the long bones are quite straight; the 'bowing' is due to lateral displacement of the posterior compartment muscles, which is due to:

- medial rotation of lower leg (medial genicular position)
- genu varum
- adaptive shortening of medial knee joint muscles and connective tissues.

Clinical tests for the lower leg

While it is feasible to examine the tibiofibular unit in all planes, it is of most clinical relevance to concentrate on the transverse plane and assess tibial torsion in comparison to genicular position (transverse plane position of tibia versus femur).

Transverse plane

True tibial (tibiofibular) torsion involves lateral axial change and occurs as a part of normal development (changes in Japanese children with respect to sitting postures; Yagi 1994). While estimates of the proportions vary, there is uniformity in observations of intoeing gait, which support this as a normally decreasing finding with age (see Ch. 10).

Tibial torsion (or position) is a common contributor to an adducted gait pattern and has been estimated to change with age as follows and as represented by the transmalleolar axis angle to the frontal (coronal) plane:

1–3% of adults:	intoe due to medial torsion
5–9% school-age children:	intoe due to medial torsion
30% of toddlers:	intoe due to medial torsion.

Transmalleolar axis:

0°	birth
6°	1 year old
10–15°	2 years old
20–30°	6–8 years old

(Cusick 1990, Fabry et al 1994; Fig. 4.11).

Recent research has questioned the degree to which tibial torsion changes with age. A French study (1319 children aged 3–10 years) found minimal change in tibial torsion: 34° at age 3 years and 36° at age 10 years (as assessed using the transmalleolar axis; Jacquemier et al 2008). A larger Chinese study (2630 children) found that tibial torsion changed from 15° at 2 years to 35° at 12 years (using the thigh–foot angle; Fabry et al 1994, Jacquemier et al 2008). Neither study found major gender variation for the development of tibial torsion.

Tibial torsion may be represented clinically as the transmalleolar axis (TMA) on the frontal plane (Fig. 4.11). TMA of 35° lateral is normally found in the adult population (Fabry et al 1994). As described by Engel and Staheli, TMA can be assessed as follows:

- child seated
- flexed knee hanging over table edge
- ankle at 90°
- measure TMA vs coronal/frontal plane.

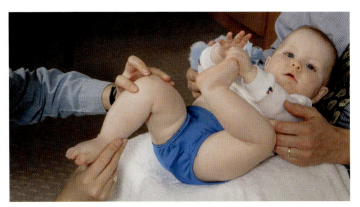

Figure 4.11 This fraught proxy for tibial torsion must be used with caution. In vivo, the distal tibia and fibular position are compared with the proximal tibia. The position of the tibial tuberosity may vary between subjects more than the position of the tibial condyles, such that it may be wise to use the latter as proximal landmarks. Important is the appreciation of bony tibial (tibiofibular) torsion from genicular position. The thigh–foot angle is a useful test to include in the assessment of the transverse plane orientation of the lower leg.

Key *Concepts*

The thigh–foot angle enables further assessment of the tibia and can be usefully compared with angle of gait (Fig. 4.12). The average thigh–foot angle is 10° abducted (Fabry et al 1994).

Ankle: talocrural joint

The ankle joint complex comprises articular facets between the tibia, talus and fibula. The primary motion provided is in the sagittal plane and the most stable position for the ankle is in dorsiflexion due to the trapezoid shape of the talar trochlear surface wedging firmly between the distal tibia and fibula.

The trochlear surface of the talus is broader anteriorly and fits more closely between the tibia and fibula (in dorsiflexion) than the posterior surface (in plantarflexion).

The malleoli spread slightly with ankle dorsiflexion, within the limits of the tibiofibular ligaments. Muscles responsible for dorsiflexion (extensors) do not attach to the fibula, allowing it to separate from the tibia with the talar 'wedging' in the ankle mortice, as occurs with dorsiflexion.

The convex trochlear surface of the talus moves beneath the concave surface of the distal tibia. In dorsiflexion the talar trochlea glides posteriorly

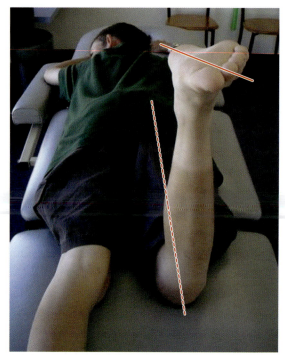

Figure 4.12 The thigh–foot angle is clinically indicative of tibial torsion/malleolar position. In this boy the thigh–foot angle approximates 20° abducted, reflecting the knee position in the transverse plane. This is a very useful test in children who intoe or outtoe appreciably, as it separates the lower and upper leg components. The thigh–foot angle needs to be compared with the angle of gait to detect the level/s of compensation.

and medially, whereas with plantarflexion the talar trochlea moves anteriorly and laterally.

The shape of the trochlear surface of the talus results in greater ankle joint mobility (and potential instability) in plantarflexion than when the joint is dorsiflexed. Plantarflexion of the ankle joint induces frontal plane motion of the talus, which in turn results in greater subtalar joint mobility.

Lateral ankle joint stability increases during development (from about the 12th gestational week) as the length of the fibula surpasses that of the tibia.

Ligamentous support holds the talus firmly within the developing ankle mortice. Muscular support of the ankle joint complex consists of:

- tibialis anterior
- triceps surae (especially soleus)
- tibialis posterior
- long extensors and flexors.

All of these muscles functionally assist stability in frontal and sagittal planes in both stance and swing phases. Contact subtalar joint pronation is accompanied by dorsiflexion of the ankle and supinatory propulsion occurs with ankle plantarflexion.

Range of motion

A large amount of motion is available in the newborn due to physiological flexion in the normal full-term gestational infant. There may be up to 70° of dorsiflexion (dorsum of foot opposing anterior tibia) and 30° of plantarflexion. In the newborn the rest position of the ankle is some 15° plantarflexed.

Hypermobility of the ankle reduces rapidly in the first few weeks of postnatal life. The initially increased ankle range of motion is due to intrauterine positioning and maternal hormones released during birth.

The passive range in the normal infant (after newborn hypermobility) is approximately 45°.

Structure of the talocrural joint and rear foot at birth

There is both confusion and disagreement among published authors as to the structure and position of the ankle joint at birth. Some describe rear foot valgus while others describe rear foot varus in the newborn (Cusick 1990, DeValentine 1992, Drennan 1992, Tachdjian 1985). The latter talk about an open kinetic chain rear foot varus which compensates to valgus in closed kinetic chain and suggest that calcaneovalgus at birth is abnormal and due to adaptive intrauterine moulding (Cusick 1990).

Further research has looked at the angle of the tibial plafond. Findings have suggested that the tibial plafond is everted in the frontal plane at birth, with development seeing it align on the frontal plane by age 12 years (Tachdjian 1985).

The fibula is relatively short (as compared to its adult fibula–tibia ratio) at birth and the increasing length does provide greater stability of the talus in the frontal plane.

Ankle equinus

Defined as reduced sagittal plane motion at the ankle mortice whilst the subtalar joint is in its neutral position (meaning less than 5–10° of available dorsiflexion).

According to Tachdjian (1985), ankle equinus exhibits the following associations:

- Contracture of the triceps surae or a disto-anterior tibial exostosis.
- Disrupted agonist/antagonist relationship of the triceps surae and tibialis anterior such that normal heel–toe gait patterns are lost.
- Common deformity of the foot and ankle in cerebral palsy, where gastrocnemius is the main proponent.
- Results in both static and functional foot and knee compensations (see Fig. 4.13).

Classification

There are four basic types of ankle equinus. These are listed in order of prevalence:

1. gastrocnemius equinus
2. gastrosoleal equinus
3. soleal equinus
4. osseous (bony block).

Key *Concepts*

Remember that the hamstrings also cross the knee joint posteriorly and may be associated with reduced extension of that joint in conjunction with gastrocnemius shortness and ligament tightness.

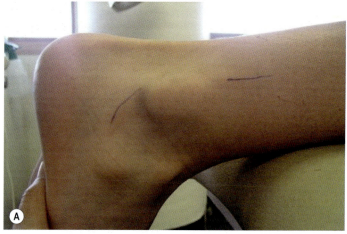

Figure 4.13 Ankle equinus (A), in addition to forefoot varus

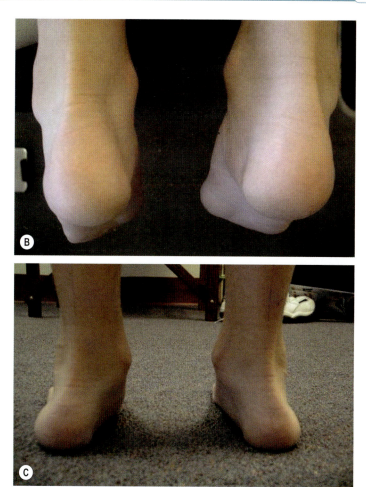

Figure 4.13 *Continued.* (B) resulting in weight-bearing compensations through the midtarsal joints/area (C) subtalar joints.

Ankle equinus is suggested to be an extremely destructive condition as far as the foot is concerned, as a result of the numerous forceful compensations it demands at many levels. Listed below are a 'top 10' of compensations/pathologies and resulting deformities clinically associated with ankle equinus:

1. genu recurvatum
2. fixed knee flexion (spastic hamstrings as in cerebral palsy)
3. rear foot/subtalar valgus
4. vertical talus → rocker bottom foot → peroneal spasm
5. forefoot supinatus → forefoot varus → hypermobile first ray
6. increased angle of gait (abducted)
7. medial protrusion of talonavicular joint
8. clawed toes
9. hallux valgus
10. toe walking.

Remember that the gastrocnemius crosses three joints (knee, ankle, subtalar) while soleus crosses two joints (ankle, subtalar). As a result it is important to test ankle range with the knee both extended and flexed (although knee flexion has been associated with unreliable measures; Evans & Scutter 2006).

Clinical testing: the concept of resistance levels

Of particular use in children with neurological impairment is the examination of muscle group resistance levels. This is a useful way of differentiating functional range from connective tissue capacity (Beenakker et al 2005, Cusick 1990, Tardieu et al 1988). Observing resistance levels (which can direct stretching programmes) can be easily incorporated into the standard ankle range examination, as follows:

Lie the child prone. Position yourself lateral to lower leg and foot, child's knee extended. Stabilize the subtalar joint ('neutral' position) to prevent pronation. Passively dorsiflex the ankle to first resistance level (= first resistance, R1). Increase passive dorsiflexion force to end resistance (= second resistance, R2).

You can also ask the child to actively assist dorsiflexion (if appropriate).

Repeat with the knee flexed.

Assess the quality of end range of motion with respect to an osseous block.

In theory, the R1 findings should be similar between practitioners, as this assesses the muscle length, ankle range. R2 will be dependent on the examiner's strength. Active dorsiflexion will vary according to children's age, neurological status, extensor strength.

Range of motion expected in the infant ankle

Children's ankle dorsiflexion can range from 20° to 50° in infants and toddlers and reduces to approximately 5–20° in adults. A range of 10° is widely regarded as the minimal requirement for normal gait function. Too little ankle dorsiflexion will disrupt the ankle rocker model, which it turn results in compensations in both the foot and more proximal leg, knee, hip (Perry 1992, Perry et al 2003).

Ankle plantarflexion ranges from 30° to 45° on average for all ages, with approximately 20° required for normal gait.

Author's note

The next sections delve into the basic biomechanics of the subtalar, midtarsal and first ray joint complexes. While clearly pertinent to the podiatrist, notable too is the fact that little research has specifically evaluated these joints in paediatric feet. What follows is a very basic coverage of these areas, necessarily derived from adult subject findings.

Subtalar joint: talocalcaneal facets

The function of the subtalar joint is to adapt the foot to transverse plane motions via the triplane motions of pronation and supination. The subtalar joint, its axis and associated motion has stood up to the scrutiny of research and investigation with greater consistency than has the midtarsal joint (Keenan 1997; Root et al 1971, 1977).

Motion about the subtalar joint occurs about an axis (as does all motion). The 'average' subtalar joint axis is located approximately 45° from the transverse plane and 15° from the sagittal plane (Root et al 1977). Axial pitch variation was acknowledged with variation in pitch from the transverse plane ranging between 20° and 60° (Kirby 1987, Root et al 1977).

Axial pitch (triplane gradient) determines the proportion of motion to occur in each plane (Fig. 4.14). If the axial pitch changes, it follows that the proportion of planal motions to occur will also alter (Fig. 4.15; Kirby 1988, 1989).

Remember that while we generally observe and measure subtalar joint range of motion on the frontal/coronal plane (inversion, eversion), this is only *representing* true subtalar joint motion, which is triplane. Understanding axial variation helps to understand the functioning of different feet in gait, e.g. a higher pitched subtalar joint axis will allow more adduction, abduction in the transverse plane. Clinically, a medial skive (Kirby 1987, 1988, 1992, 2001) will be more useful than basic rear foot posting in limiting subtalar pronation range/speed in this foot type – hence better orthotic prescription is availed from understanding axial positions and the functional ramifications.

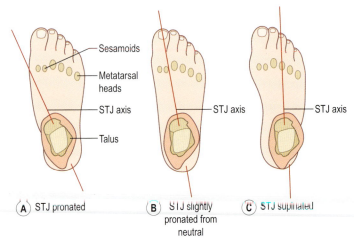

Figure 4.14 Clinically, this depicts the axial shift or variation of the subtalar joint (STJ) axis in different foot types and the ground response in supinating or pronating the foot about its axis. (A) Most ground reaction force is lateral to the axis, pronating the foot throughout gait and in stance. There is reduced area to place a supinatory force medial to the STJ axis, which is relevant to both footwear and orthotic selection. (B) Ground reaction forces will equilibrate about the axis, promoting a normal gait pattern and stance. (C) More ground reaction force is medial to the axis, supinating the foot throughout gait and in stance. This is the typical foot type associated with ankle inversion sprains. Posting this foot at the lateral forefoot can improve re-supination into propulsion very effectively.

Landmarks for location of subtalar joint neutral position

Theoretically, the subtalar joint (STJ) neutral position is defined as being the position where the STJ is neither pronated nor supinated – it is, if you like, a *cusp* position.

Traditional teaching instructed three methods and associated sets of anatomical landmarks to locate the neutral position of the subtalar joint:

- talonavicular joint congruity
- lateral malleolar depressions
- 'arc' of joint motion (point from which motion direction changes).

Clearly the arc of motion is not applicable in the closed kinetic chain examination.

Rear foot developmental changes

At birth the subtalar joint has a varus attitude to the leg (approximately 10°). At 12 months of age the calcaneus rests at approximately 10°

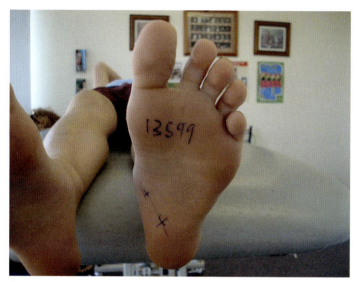

Figure 4.15 This boy has a medially positioned subtalar joint axis, which is determined from palpating the plantar surface and noting the inversion/plantarflexion versus the eversion/dorsiflexion of the fourth to fifth metatarsal heads. Clinically this method is very helpful in determining the placement of orthotic skives or posting. Clinically it can be useful to apply adhesive felt wedging to the plantar aspect of the patient's foot and then observe their stance and gait to ensure positioning medial to the subtalar axis (and the required gait effect).

everted in closed kinetic chain due to compensation for this open kinetic chain varus. The resting calcaneal stance position reduces with age over the first 6–8 years of life (Drennan 1992, Tachdjian 1985).

Midtarsal joint

Traditionally the midtarsal joint was regarded as consisting of the talonavicular and calcaneocuboid joints. More recently the calcaneonavicular and cuboid-navicular joints have also been considered to be part of this functional complex.

Traditional theory tells us that the midtarsal joint functions to minimize transverse plane forces between ground and leg (Root et al 1977). The two axes model predominated until the late 1990s and has since been deposed (Keenan 1997). More recent research has proposed a single axis model, complementary to the cardinal body planes (Nestor & Findlow 2006). You will need to modify your understanding as more research findings become available.

The new single axis model for the midtarsal joint

The contemporary model for the midtarsal joint proposes motion about one axis of rotation and uses both global and local 3-D coordinates defined within the cardinal body planes (Fig. 4.16). In essence, this model reduces much of the previous complexity by regarding the talonavicular and calcaneocuboid joints as one 'block' segment, which moves relative to the calcaneus segment. With the single axis model, all motion is observed and described about three reference axes (Table 4.2).

The axes are defined around the medial, lateral and posterior aspects of the calcaneus. This model standardizes the reference planes for motion about the midtarsal joint as already occurs for the ankle, subtalar and first ray joints and better links clinical foot assessment with research modelling and discussion (Nestor & Findlow 2006).

Clinical assessment of the midtarsal joint

Practically in assessing the midtarsal joint we are trying to compare the transverse plane of the forefoot with the transverse plane of the rear foot (Fig. 4.17) and measure the angle between them. There are some 'rules' to abide by in this exercise:

- subtalar joint placed in 'neutral'
- dorsiflex fourth and fifth rays to 'lock' midtarsal joint on the subtalar joint
- observe/measure the forefoot plane compared to the rear foot plane
- determine forefoot varus/valgus (with forefoot valgus, differentiate from possible plantarflexion of the first ray).

The reliability of assessment of the midtarsal joint (forefoot to rear foot relationship) has been found to be inversely proportional to age (Table 4.3); hence this measure/observation is of little use in young children (Evans et al 2003).

Midtarsal joint developmental changes

At birth the newborn forefoot is inverted 10–15° on the rear foot. This position has been described as embryonic 'praying' (see Ch. 2). Postnatal development sees the non-weight-bearing forefoot varus (or its soft tissue component of *supinatus*) maintained by:

- shortened medial soft tissues
- possibly, talar torsion.

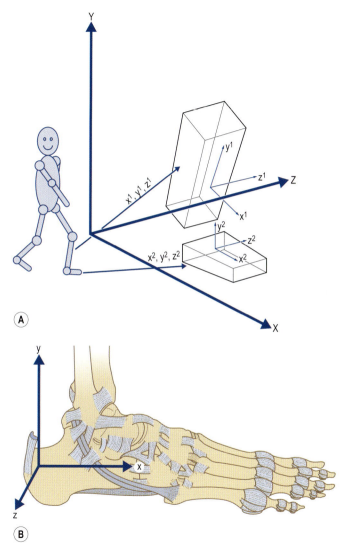

Figure 4.16 (A) The single axis midtarsal joint model. As seen, the axis is plotted in 3-D by x, y and z coordinates; x coordinate: inversion/eversion, y coordinate: abduction/adduction, z coordinate: plantarflexion/dorsiflexion.
(B) This model conceptually regards the midtarsal joint as that between the calcaneus and the 'block' of the talonavicular/calcaneocuboid joints.

Table 4.2

Axis	Orientation	Cardinal planes	Motion
x	Anterior/posterior	Transverse, sagittal	Frontal plane
y	Superior/inferior	Sagittal, frontal	Transverse plane
z	Medial/lateral	Frontal, transverse	Sagittal plane

Table 4.3

Subject age (years)	Reliability (inter-rater ICC)
4–6	0.28
8–15	0.53
20–50	0.70

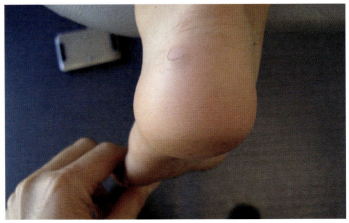

Figure 4.17 The clinical midtarsal joint forefoot–rear foot relationship of forefoot varus.

Talar torsion is the lateral twist through the talar head and neck and may also include adduction (Cusick 1990, Drennan 1992, Tachdjian 1985).

First ray complex: medial cuneiform and first metatarsal

The axis of the first ray has the opposite orientation to those of the more proximal subtalar and midtarsal joints. The axis angles between 10–20°

from the transverse plane in children and 15–30° from the transverse plane in adults. It deviates 50° from the sagittal plane (Cusick 1990).

The first ray axis allows dorsiflexion and inversion (slight adduction) with closed kinetic chain pronation and plantarflexion and eversion (slight abduction) with closed kinetic chain supination.

The longitudinal bisection of the first ray approximately parallels that of the talus (from the transverse plane; Valmassy 1996).

The motion of the first ray is primarily dorsiflexion and plantarflexion, secondly abduction and adduction, and least is inversion and eversion.

Clinical assessment of first ray motion and position

Again there are 'rules' to follow, similar to those for the midtarsal joint examination.

Place subtalar joint in neutral position and ' lock'/pronate the midtarsal joint. Hold metatarsal heads two to five with one hand and the first metatarsal head with the opposite hand. Dorsiflex and plantarflex the first metatarsal head through its sagittal plane range of motion, while stabilizing the lesser metatarsals with the other hand. Observe the proportion of the available ranges of motion in terms of dorsiflexion and plantarflexion:

– dorsiflexion > plantarflexion = dorsiflexed first ray
– dorsiflexion < plantarflexion = plantarflexed first ray (rigid/flexible)
– dorsiflexion = plantarflexion = neutral first ray

(knowing the thickness of your thumbs is useful when observing this range).

Check the first metatarsophalangeal joint range of motion:

– 65–75° is required for functional toe-off stability.

Summary

Key Concepts

> Developmental biomechanics as affecting the lower limb can be regarded as a gradual unwinding process, which facilitates extension, strengthening and activation of the hip, thigh, leg and foot.

While precise values vary, there is good agreement between authors and research investigation over many years, which concur on the following 12 points:

1. The initially flexed spine develops cervical and lumbar lordoses.
2. Hip range of motion is initially greater lateral than medial (approximate ratio 2 : 1), equalizing by age 2–3 years.

3. Femoral torsion at birth approximates 40° medial and reduces to 10° by skeletal maturity. Values are approximately 10° less in males than females.

4. Genu varum is present at birth, but abnormal after 2 years of age.

5. Genu valgum reaches maximum value by age 4 years, approximating 10°.

6. Tibial torsion is probably minimal at birth and reaches 20° by age 8 years (as imaged by CT).

7. Transmalleolar axis approximates 35° lateral (NB: the values for tibial torsion and TMA are the most disparate across reported findings).

8. Thigh–foot angle ranges from adducted 10° to abducted 20° at age 2 years and reaches approximately 20–30° abducted by ages 8–10 years.

9. Ankle dorsiflexion reduces from approximately 40° in the newborn with 5–10° remaining for normal gait.

10. The rear foot is inverted some 10° to the lower leg at birth, giving rise to an initial weight-bearing heel eversion angle (RCSP) of 10°. This reduces to vertical/slight eversion by 6–8 years.

11. The forefoot is inverted relative to the rear foot in utero and reduces until approximately 6–8 years.

12. Altered muscle tone (as with cerebral palsy) and increased ligament laxity are associated with variation from normative values for age.

References

Accadbled F, Laville J-M, Harper L 2003 One-step treatment for evolved Blount's disease. Journal of Pediatric Orthopedics 23(6):747–752

Beenakker EAC, Fock JM, Van Tol MJ et al 2005 Intermittent prednisone therapy in Duchenne muscular dystrophy: a randomized controlled trial. Archives of Neurology 62(1):128–132

Beeson P 1999 Frontal plane configuration of the knee in children. The Foot 9:18–26

Cheng JCY, Chan PS, Chiang SC 1991 Angular and rotational profile of the lower limb in 2630 Chinese children. Journal of Pediatric Orthopedics 11(2):154–161

Colson ER, Levenson S, Rybin D et al 2006 Barriers to following the supine sleep recommendation among mothers at four centers for the women, infants, and children program. Pediatrics 118(2):e243–e250

Cusick BD 1990 Progressive casting and splinting for lower extermity deformities in children with neuromotor dysfunction. Therapy Skill Builders, Arizona

Cusick BD, Stuberg WA 1992 Assessment of lower-extremity alignment in the transverse plane: implications for management of children with neuromotor dysfunction. Physical Therapy 72(1):13–25

Davids JR, Benfanti P, Blackhurst DW et al 2002 Assessment of femoral anteversion in children with cerebral palsy: accuracy of the trochanteric prominence angle test. Journal of Pediatric Orthopedics 22(2):173–178

Deeg KH, Lode HM, Gassner I 2007 Spinal sonography in newborns and infants. Part I: Method, normal anatomy and indications. Ultraschall in der Medizin 28(5):507–517

DeValentine SJ 1992 Foot and ankle disorders in children. Churchill Livingstone, New York

Drennan JC 1992 The child's foot and ankle. Raven Press, New York

Eckhoff DG, Johnson KK 1994 Three-dimensional computed tomography reconstruction of tibial torsion. Clinical Orthopedics 302:64–68

Evans AM, Scutter S 2006 Sagittal plane range of motion of the pediatric ankle joint. a reliability study. Journal of the American Podiatric Medical Association 96(5):418–422

Evans AM, Copper AW, Scharfbillig RW et al 2003 Reliability of the foot posture index and traditional measures of foot position. Journal of the American Podiatric Medical Association 93(3):203

Fabry G, Cheng LX, Molenaers G 1994 Normal and abnormal torsional development in children. Clinical Orthopaedics and Related Research (302):22–26

Glenn OA, Barkovich J 2006 Magnetic resonance imaging of the fetal brain and spine: an increasingly important tool in prenatal diagnosis. Part 2. AJNR American Journal of Neuroradiology 27(9):1807–1814

Guidera KJ, Ganey TM, Keneally CR et al 1994 The embryology of lower-extremity torsion. Clinical Orthopaedics and Related Research (302):17–21

Heath CH, Staheli LT 1993 Normal limits of knee angle in white children – genu varum and genu valgum. Journal of Pediatric Orthopedics 13(2):259–262

Jacquemier M, Glard Y, Pomero V et al 2008 Rotational profile of the lower limb in 1319 healthy children. Gait and Posture 28(2):187–193

Keenan A-M 1997 A clinician's guide to the practical implications of the recent controversy of foot function. Australasian Journal of Podiatric Medicine 31(3):87–93

Kirby KA 1987 Methods for determination of positional variations in the subtalar joint axis. Journal of the American Podiatric Medical Association 77(5):228

Kirby KA 1988 Anterior axial projection of the foot. Journal of the American Podiatric Medical Association 78(7):380b

Kirby KA 1989 Rotational equilibrium across the subtalar joint axis. Journal of the American Podiatric Medical Association 79(1):1

Kirby KA 1992 The medial heel skive technique. Improving pronation control in foot orthoses. Journal of the American Podiatric Medical Association 82(4):177

Kirby KA 2001 Subtalar joint axis location and rotational equilibrium theory of foot function. Journal of the American Podiatric Medical Association 91(9):465

Kumar SJ, MacEwen GD 1982 Torsional abnormalities in children's lower extremities. Orthopedic Clinics of North America 13(3):629–639

Lang LMG, Volpe RG 1998 Measurement of tibial torsion. Journal of the American Podiatric Medical Association 88(4):160–165

Lowe LH, Johanek AJ, Moore CW 2007 Sonography of the neonatal spine. Part 1: Normal anatomy, imaging pitfalls, and variations that may simulate disorders. American Journal of Roentgenology 188(3): 733–738

Mac-Thiong JM, Berthonnaud E, Dimar JR et al 2004 Sagittal alignment of the spine and pelvis during growth. Spine 29(15):1642–1647

Moon RY, Oden RP, Grady KC 2004 Back to sleep: an educational intervention with women, infants, and children program clients. Pediatrics 113(3):542–547

Nestor CJ, Findlow AH 2006 Clinical and experimental models of the midtarsal joint. Journal of the American Podiatric Medical Association 96(1):24–31

Pasciak M, Stoll TM, Hefti F 1996 Relation of femoral to tibial torsion in children measured by ultrasound. Journal of Pediatric Orthopedics B 5(4):268–272

Perry JP 1992 Gait analysis: normal and pathological function. Slack, Thorofare, NJ

Perry J, Burnfield JM, Gronley JK et al 2003 Toe walking: muscular demands at the ankle and knee. Archives of Physical Medicine and Rehabilitation 84:7–16

Root ML, Orien WP, Weed JH et al 1971 Biomechanical examination of the foot. Clinical Biomechanics Corporation, Los Angeles

Root ML, Weed JH, Orien WP 1977 Normal and abnormal function of the foot. Clinical Biomechanics Corporation, Los Angeles

Schneider B, Laubenberger J, Jemlich S et al 1997 Measurement of femoral antetorsion and tibial torsion by magnetic resonance imaging. British Journal of Radiology 70(834):575–579

Shacklock M 2005 Clinical neurodynamics. Elsevier, London

Shepherd RB 1995 Physiotherapy in paediatrics, 3rd edn. Butterworth Heinemann, Oxford

Staheli LT 1989 Torsion: treatment considerations. Clinical Orthopaedics and Related Research (247):61–66

Stein-Zamir C, Volovik I, Rishpon S et al 2008 Developmental dysplasia of the hip: risk markers, clinical screening and outcome. Pediatrics International 50(3):341–345

Tachdjian MO 1985 The child's foot. WB Saunders, Philadelphia

Tardieu C, Lespargot A, Tabary C et al 1988 For how long must the soleus muscle be stretched each day to prevent contracture? Developmental Medicine and Child Neurology 30(1):3–10

Valmassy RL 1996 Clinical biomechanics of the lower extremities. Mosby, St Louis, p. 246

Yagi T 1994 Tibial torsion in patients with medial type osteoarthritic knees. Clinical Orthopaedics and Related Research (302):52–56

Further reading

Cusick BD 1990 Progressive casting and splinting for lower extremity deformities in children with neuromotor dysfunction. Therapy Skill Builders, Arizona

DeValentine SJ 1992 Foot and ankle disorders in children. Churchill Livingstone, New York

Drennan JC 1992 The child's foot and ankle. Raven Press, New York

Tachdjian MO 1985 The child's foot. WB Saunders, Philadelphia

Tachdjian, MO 1997 Clinical pediatric orthopedics: the art of diagnosis and principles of management. Appleton & Lange, Stamford, CT

Watkins J 2009 Pocket podiatry. Functional anatomy. Elsevier, Oxford

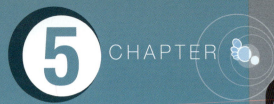

5 CHAPTER

Gait development

Introduction

Gait analysis in the clinical setting is a valuable part of decision making when initially assessing a child and when reviewing their progress and the effects of any treatments. Normal paediatric gait is complex, but abnormal gait is even more complex as seen in children with cerebral palsy. These children are best assessed with 3-D motion measurement in a gait laboratory, as this gives best diagnosis and therapeutic planning, be this surgical or orthotic in nature. However, the clinician must be able to observe gait simply and make qualitative judgements about a child's gait based on the visual appearance and noting the following factors:

- balance
- stability
- speed
- movement control
- symmetry
- limb and trunk motion
- weight transfer
- foot type and placement.

(Rose et al 1991).

Observation gives valuable information about a child's overall walking pattern and their ability to function. Video gait analysis can be useful to review features without the child being present and to save protracted gait observation.

Key *Concepts*

> The clinician should be aware that gait on a treadmill is usually quite different to normal gait and observed gait may differ from usual gait. The use of a walkway is therefore recommended.

The history of gait analysis began in Europe in the 17th century and continues to evolve and embellish our current understanding of human walking (Sutherland 2001, 2002). Sutherland has been one of the notable contemporary investigators of paediatric gait, in association with many other prominent scientists, and the reader is directed to this work for greater understanding of this area (Cusick 1990; Gage 1993; Perry 1992; Rose et al 1991; Sutherland 1978, 2001, 2002).

Paediatric gait and stance

We need to remember that human bipedal walking is preceded by a number of necessary preparatory stages (Cusick 1990).

Key *Concepts*

> The basic antigravity skills adopted in both prone and supine floor positions are essential in the development of the infant's ability to extend and flex joints, lengthen muscles and attain the agonist–antagonist relationship which promotes normal bony modelling and movement patterns (Figs 5.1 and 5.2).

What follows is a summary of the landmark stages in gait development with reference to age-related trends. Note that many of these stages are by definition 'pre-walking'. The vast realm of pathological gait is largely outside this modest account and the reader is advised to look at the Further reading section at the end of this chapter, and beyond, for deeper understanding and further detail.

The neurodevelopmental progress of newborn term infants is checked routinely by paediatricians at 6 weeks of age. At this time, a reduction in flexor tone of the limbs is observed, together with an increase in active neck tone. Visual orientation improves by 3 weeks when normal infants can follow a target in a full circle compared to newborns that are often only able to follow a target in an arc. Research results suggest that 6 weeks post-term birth is an important milestone for changes in neurological signs, particularly those related to muscle tone and posture, which reflect maturation of the nervous system (Guzzetta et al 2005).

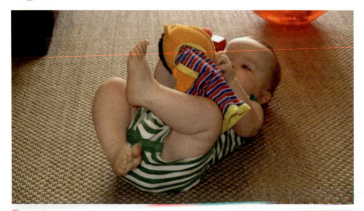

Figure 5.1 Supine floor play promotes extension of hips and knees, reducing the physiological flexion seen in the newborn. The increasing weight of the limbs with growth facilitates 'baby weight training' which builds strength and coordinates movements.

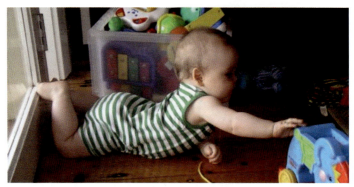

Figure 5.2 Prone floor play sees active extension and promotes the development of both cervical and lumbar lordoses. The neck muscles have attained very good strength and control to lift the head. This child shows a well-controlled propping of the upper body with his left arm while reaching and extending his right arm to reach/push the toy.

Sitting

Sitting is a real landmark in the child's development and is usually accomplished by approximately 6 months of age. Sitting indicates that the child has attained enough strength in the neck, trunk and hip extensors to be able to hold a raised head position against gravity while maintaining a sitting position on a stable pelvis. The legs and feet are usually in front of the child. The legs are laterally rotated and the feet abducted. This position (sometimes called 'ring sitting') provides good stability against forward or lateral falling. However, the new sitter is prone to falling backwards, which is why experienced parents, grandparents and miscellaneous caregivers rush to place pillows behind the novice sitter. When the child has learned to balance their extension and flexion, they can begin to introduce both lateral and rotating movements (Fig. 5.3).

The evident pattern of movement development at this stage is to be repeated in the development of later gait phases; i.e. sagittal plane motions:

- precede frontal plane motions
- precede transverse plane motions.

Abnormal sitting where the child sags back onto their sacrum may occur in children with spastic diplegia. In these children, there is lack of trunk extension strength, inadequate hip joint mobility and shortness of hamstrings, adductors and abdominals. These children will have to compensate for their lack of available movement ranges and develop irregular gait patterns. Hypotonia may also be associated with seated 'sagging' but is usually associated with normal to increased hip range.

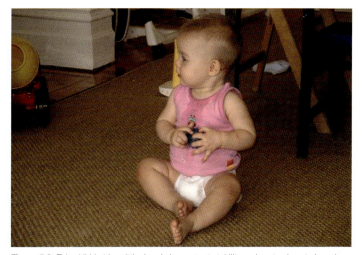

Figure 5.3 This child is 'ring sitting' and shows great stability and postural control as she also manages to play with a ball and look across to her mother. Note the full extension of the neck and trunk, yet the remaining lower limb flexion.

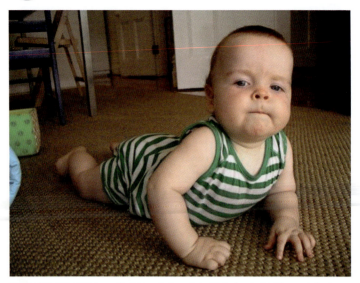

Figure 5.4 This child has gained enough strength to lift his head, shoulders and chest. Pulling with his arms and pushing forward along the floor with his feet facilitates movement, especially gluteal activity, and hip/leg extension.

'Ring sitting' posture provides the stability from which a child can lean forward into a three-point vault and eventually creep on all fours. The child usually tummy crawls around 5 months of age when they 'swim' prone and exercise good spine and hip/knee extension (Fig. 5.4).

Creeping

From the lower limb perspective, active weight-bearing and rocking motions on hands and knees strengthens and stabilizes the hips, deepening the pelvic acetabular cups. Coupled eccentric and concentric contractions around shoulders and hips prevent the infant from falling forward and onto their face by initiating a backward shift. Pelvic support is essential at this stage and requires abdominal muscle efficiency.

Creeping usually follows from playing where a child will reach and lean and diagonally load the non-reaching side. Stability of the loaded side is required and the adductors stabilize the loaded hip. Reciprocal creeping occurs as an extension of this unilateral reach and lean, where each side takes its turn. Learned proficiency and maturity of the neuromotor struc-

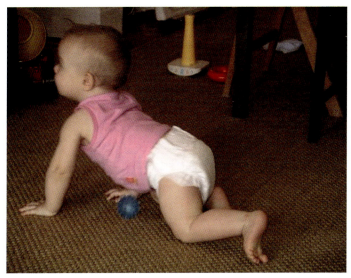

Figure 5.5 This child has progressed from tummy crawling to being quadriped on hands and knees. She has gained enough strength and postural control to be able to lift and carry her trunk off the floor. Weighting the shoulders and hips assists the stability and coordination of these joints. The left leg is extending, producing a torque to reduce femoral torsion and increase tibial torsion.

tures mean the child will narrow their quad-base of support (as later occurs with bipedal walking) and develop counter-rotations between shoulders and pelvis (as also occurs with maturity of the later walking pattern).

Reciprocal creeping appears to apply a lateral torque to the pushing side femur above an extending knee and laterally rotating hip (Fig. 5.5). Adductor magnus acts to stabilize the hip and in so doing contributes to the torque force through the femur, which in turn reduces femoral torsion (approximately 40° medial at birth and 'unwinding' 25% in the first 24 months).

Some children do not creep properly, preferring to 'bottom shuffle' along in a sitting position. This may be due to hypotonia which results in inadequate stabilizing of shoulders and pelvis, or may be associated with sensory integration and result from tactile defensiveness. Examination and wider history taking will usually distinguish low muscle tone from noxious sensory input by elucidating some key factors, e.g.:

	Hypotonia	Sensory integration
Concept	– less neural impulses/time to muscles	– noxious experience of (normal) sensory stimuli
Clinical signs	– sluggish tendon reflexes – flaccid feel of muscle bellies – late motor milestones	– recoil from touch, e.g. feeding, cuddling, dressing, towel drying – more prone to toe walking (see Ch. 11) – may require desensitizing (paediatric occupational and physiotherapy)

Propping and bear-standing

Knee extension develops both supinc (babies like to play with and 'eat' their feet, which extends the knee) and prone positions. There must be good balance control, pelvis and shoulder stability to achieve this posture, which reduces physiological flexion of the lower limbs as follows:

- elongates hamstrings
- elongates triceps surae
- elongates plantar fascia and intrinsic foot muscles
- hyperextends toes (Fig. 5.6).

Kneeling

As a natural 'flop back' position from moving ('creeping') on all fours, the position of knee-sitting arises at around 8 months of age. With variation of this position to side sitting and full sitting, much stability of the hips is required to control lateral and rotating positions. The trunk is lengthened and strengthened and there are forces applied increasingly to develop the femoral greater trochanter (gluteus medius activity) and proximal femoral torsion 'unwinding', which contribute to the simultaneous reductions in medial femoral torsion and position (antetorsion and anteversion) (Fig. 5.7; see Ch. 4).

Kneel-sit to kneel-stand positions also reduce femoral torsion by extending hip flexors and mobilizing the anterior hip capsule and ligaments. This also reduces coxa valga by applying force to the abducted femur through the gluteals (especially gluteus medius).

'W' sitting (reverse tailor's position) lowers the pelvis to the floor between the legs and may be seen in children with and without neuro-motor problems. These children may show high/age medial femoral torsion (determined clinically using Ryder's test; Cusick & Stuberg 1992)

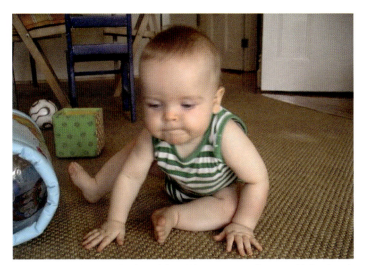

Figure 5.6 This child is moving forward from sitting to momentarily prop on his hands and right foot while he frees his left leg. This motion requires great precision and control of shifting loads. Adequate strength is needed and balance responses are practised and learned.

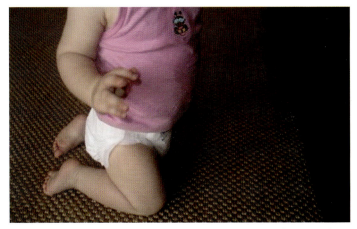

Figure 5.7 This child kneels while reaching with her left hand (not seen) for a toy on the sofa. Note the simultaneous trunk rotation and the right arm extension to counterbalance this skilful manoeuvre.

and which is often familial ('I used to sit like that too' says a parent, with retained femoral torsion). According to Staheli (Fuchs & Staheli 1996, Staheli 1987), children with normal muscle tone and increased medial femoral torsion show no limitation of athletic or functional ability. There may, however, be compensation at the knee via greater lateral genicular rotation (Staheli 1987; Fig. 5.8) and patella maltracking, which is apparent as a part of symptomatic patellofemoral syndrome (Beaty 1993).

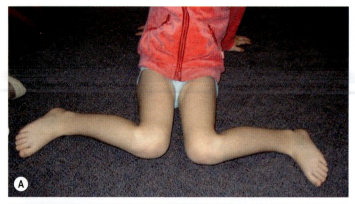

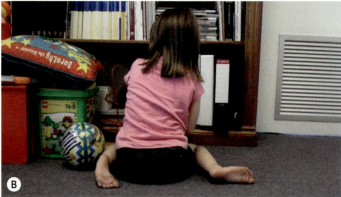

Figure 5.8 The key suspicions in older children who continue to W sit are medial hip position and non-resolving femoral torsion. The lower legs may be positioned symmetrically or not, which often pairs with stance and foot angles in gait (A) Child A showed medial knee positions in gait, but straight feet. (B) Child B displayed left adduction and right abduction in gait.

W sitting is a common compensation for children with neuromotor problems of either hypotonia or hypertonia. Cusick (1990) states that after 2 years of age, W sitting reveals and exaggerates medial torsion in the femoral shaft, i.e. femoral torsion fails to reduce physiologically, in effect retaining an osseous '*immaturity*'. Children with higher degrees of medial femoral torsion are more likely to W sit, which in turn may affect (retard) the expected reduction in femoral torsion. The W sitting position is often used by children who require greater stability as it provides a wider base of seated support. If this is the only position used for floor activities the soft tissues will adapt, as may the osseous structures. Feet may be laterally rotated, medially rotated, or one of each. The proximal knee joint is where the effect of such persistent rotations is occurring, in addition to the shaft axes of the long leg bones.

Clinically there is often uneven length of the hamstrings (semimembranosus and semitendinosus are usually tight in comparison to biceps femoris, but this varies) and genicular range is greater medially than laterally when transverse rotations are observed. In some cases there will be no available lateral rotation range at the knee (i.e. the foot cannot be passively abducted relative to the knee joint midpoint) and all available range is found to be medial biased with the foot position being increasingly adducted from the knee. This relationship of the tibia and femur is termed *medial genicular bias* and is frequently confused with medial tibial torsion (see Ch. 4). The discrimination of medial genicular bias (soft tissue) and tibial torsion (osseous) is important with respect to diagnosis in the young intoeing child and clearly important in terms of management (see Ch. 9).

Cruising

This can be natural (e.g. around furniture), or assisted (with carer help). If assisted, the child usually cruises on their feet with arm support earlier than if not assisted in any way.

The child pulls to a standing posture by extending both knees. The child must redistribute their centre of gravity to do this until the quadriceps become stronger. For a while, the child who pulls to stand may not be able to sit from this position without help, as it takes time for flexion to equal the forces of extension, which develop first (Fig. 5.9; Shepherd 1995).

Cruising uses the strength that the child developed through floor play to maintain an upright position while moving. This provides preparation for unsupported standing and then walking. Simultaneously, cruising is

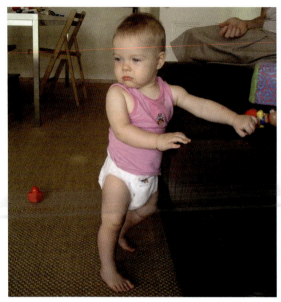

Figure 5.9 From kneeling, this child pulled-to-stand against the sofa. Note the full extension of hip and knee and ankle dorsiflexion. The left foot is placed to widen to base of support while the child rotates head and trunk to watch her sister's activities.

strengthening the limbs for bipedal weight-bearing and providing sensory input for balance and proprioception.

Climbing

Climbing is another important pre-ambulatory skill which teaches the child to disassociate their limbs. The power of the antigravity hip extensors and flexors allows the child to climb from a standing position where they exhibit supported balance. This alternating side-to-side stability and then mobility of the hips is also important in terms of reduction of femoral torsion via concentric and eccentric muscle loads (Cusick 1990). Balance, strength, agility, environment and physical confidence are other factors which may influence climbing capability.

Squatting

Squatting is usually a transition from standing to sitting, while the quadriceps are getting stronger and hamstrings have lengthened from the original state of physiological flexion. The ankle dorsiflexors activate as a counterbalance mechanism to prevent the child from toppling backwards (Fig. 5.10) and upper limbs may also be used to stabilize the trunk while learning to squat. Active ankle dorsiflexion is important for the prevention of toe drag during swing phase and decelerated forefoot loading from heel contact as gait progresses.

Standing

The newborn baby 'stands' as a part of the primitive support reflex. The same infant will also 'walk' if tilted forward as part of the stepping reflex. The primitive reflexes are of great interest, giving rise to initial activity which usually disappears or modulates before voluntary control begins (Illingworth 1987). Studies of stepping behaviour of infants show consistency in weight acceptance with a period of *astasia* (refusal to stand) occurring transiently in some children between 2 and 3 months of age. Paediatricians and neurologists assess the newborn's reflexive behaviour to assess neurological status. Developmental progress assessment will include review of the primitive reflexes, with most disappearing between 2 and 4 months of age (e.g. Moro, grasp, walking reflex) as normal development ensues. The normal baby is born with the automatic

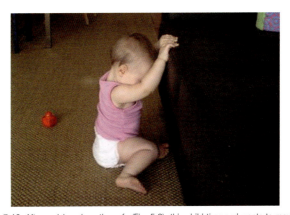

Figure 5.10 After cruising along the sofa (Fig. 5.9), this child tires and wants to move across the room to where her sister is playing. She can do this competently on all fours, but must first lower herself to the floor. Stabilizing with her hands and taking some weight through the arms, there is controlled activity of the quadriceps and triceps surae into the squat position.

('reflexive') motor patterns of stepping and walking, which become latent as limb mass increases prior to adequate muscle strength. Volitional control occurs once adequate strength is developed to initiate the motor patterns of heavier limbs (Payne & Isaacs 2008).

Key Concepts

The foot/plantar grasp reflex should be appreciated by podiatrists as it has been found to be a sensitive indicator of neurological development. In the normal infant the foot grasp reflex will be present until 2–3 months of age. It should be symmetrical and not protracted (Fig. 5.11).

Diminished or absence of the plantar grasp reflex in early infancy (up to 6 months) has been found to highly associated with neurological abnormality (especially cerebral palsy; Futagi et al 1999, Zafeiriou 2004).

The physical appearance of the foot when a normal child begins to stand will include an everted heel and a low medial longitudinal arch. Both of these features are developmentally normal and should reduce with age such that the heel is less everted and the arch becomes more apparent. A rough clinical rule-of-thumb of mine is that the initial heel eversion (resting calcaneal stance position) is less than or equal to 10° and the medial border of the foot is flat and straight in the new walking child. Heel eversion exceeding 10° and convexity of the medial border are unusual findings and need to be well assessed, monitored and, if necessary, managed. Hypermobility (associated with ligament laxity or hypotonia) is

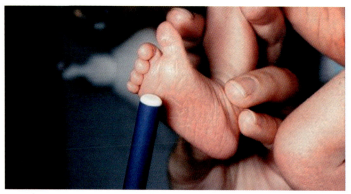

Figure 5.11 This simple but sensitive clinical test can detect neurological abnormality in infants less than 6 months of age. It should be performed gently and bilaterally. In the very small foot, a pen may be used instead of an examiner's relatively large hands.

a common association, with calcaneo-valgus posture, cerebral palsy, Down's syndrome and vertical talus (rocker-bottom foot) being other diagnostic considerations.

Gait

It is important to appreciate that the age range of walking commencement in normal children approximates 10–16 months (Ho et al 2000, Payne & Isaacs 2008). Many parents are concerned when their child is not walking by their first birthday and in most cases this is unwarranted. (It continues to amaze me, when taking a case history, just how many infants do actually begin to walk on their first birthday.) Parental expectations and culture may influence walking age by a month or two and children who are actively 'coached' to walk often do walk earlier (Shepherd 1995).

The alignment of the feet and legs in standing influences stability and resulting movement skills. The impact of poor weight-bearing skills is very obvious in children with cerebral palsy, where poor trunk stability and leg and foot positions compensating around hypertonic muscles cause reduced weight-bearing stability and functional gait.

As children's strength, balance and motor coordination improve, basic walking gait and more advanced gait patterns such as running, jumping and hopping emerge. Many potential problems with foot and leg alignment become more obvious at this time as weight-bearing and associated compensations can become functionally obvious. As a result, this is the age when parents often become concerned and seek advice. The podiatrist who sees children must have a full working knowledge of normal developmental features so that queries can be sifted and any concerns addressed.

Table 5.1 summarizes gait development with respect to age. On average girls exhibit a more mature motor developmental level, approximately 6 months ahead of boys (Payne & Isaacs 2008).

The new walking foot

An infant's early walking is characterized by short, fast, robotic steps about a wide base of support. Placing the feet wide apart helps the child to balance. This width of the base of support narrows as balance improves and after 4–5 months of independent walking the base of gait approximates trunk width (Payne & Isaacs 2008).

The arms are carried in a 'high guard' position for extra stability and arm swing is initially absent. As balance improves the arms lower and later swing in opposition to leg swing action.

Table 5.1

	Payne & Isaacs 2008	Shepherd 1995
	Age of onset	
Walking	9–17 months	From 9 months
Running	18–19 months (or 6 months after onset of walking)	18 months
Jumping	2 years	2–3 years
Single leg standing	–	4 years
Hopping	4 years	5 years
Skipping	6–7 years	–
Heel strike, walking	22 weeks after walking onset	18 months
Knee flexion, walking	–	2 months from walking onset
Adult pattern	3 years (2–6 years)	5 years

The child shows a flat-footed ground strike, rather than the later heel–toe pattern, which is seen between 18 and 24 months.

The initial angle of foot progression varies, but is usually one of decreasing abduction. However, it is not unusual to see a mild adduction or intoeing in the new walker (Cusick 1990, Ho et al 2000). More importantly, the angle of gait should be seen to be largely symmetrical, not exaggerated intoe which might cause tripping and falls and not exaggerated out-toe by foot postures such as calcaneovalgus (Fixsen & Valman 1981, Valmassy 1996).

The 1-year-old child has a relaxed calcaneal stance eversion approximating 5–10°. The child with ligamentous laxity, hypotonia or spastic diplegia may exhibit eversion of 15–30°. As a result the forefoot abducts and dorsiflexes, the toes are seen to deviate laterally and weight is taken through the medial midtarsal region. This loads the medial supporting ligaments and reduces muscle leverage of tibialis anterior and posterior to assist with tarsal stability by synergy with the peroneals. If this continues it is common to see later physiological adaptation with shortening of peroneals, lateral structures and also the triceps surae that can induce ankle equinus (Fig. 5.12).

At 2 years there is early response to weight shift via foot pronation and supination with muscle activity of the respective muscle groups. The child has lowered their arms to their sides and shows a narrowed base of gait. The child walks faster and takes longer steps due to greater strength and early signs of propulsion.

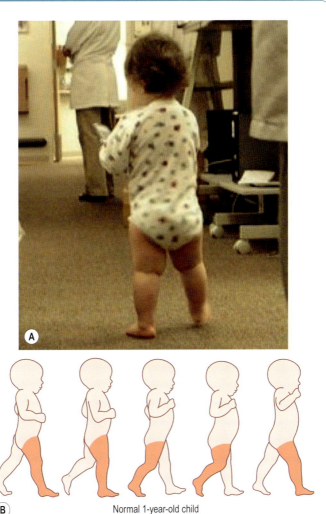

Normal 1-year-old child

Figure 5.12 (A) Stance and gait of the 1-year-old child in two planes. (B) The frontal/coronal plane shows a wide base of gait, flexed elbows and no arm swing. The sagittal plane shows one complete gait cycle/step for the right side. There is reduced hip extension which shortens the stride and the arms are held in 'high guard' for better balance. Gait maturity includes transverse plane rotation, longer strides and lowered arm swing – features which improve energy efficiency and speed.

Key Concepts

Charcot–Marie–Tooth disease (CMT)

CMT is the most common neuromuscular disorder in children, with an incidence of approximately 1 in 2500 (Charcot–Marie–Tooth Association of Australia 2008). There are some 52 identified types of CMT, with type 1A affecting some 70% of cases. CMT type 1A is genetically located on chromosome 17 and due to its progressive demyelinating effects is associated with foot and gait problems in children.

Pes cavus is the cardinal but not invariable sign of CMT 1A (Gallardo et al 2006). Other signs include:

- prominence of the fifth metatarsal styloid process
- retracted, non-weight-bearing toes, e.g. fifth
- rear foot and ankle varus (ankle sprains)
- foot drop.

Clinically, consider CMT if a child exhibits:

- pes cavus
- absent ankle reflexes
- inability to walk on their heels (expected from 2 years; Burns et al 2009, Rose et al 2008).

Inability to walk on heels has been found to be a sensitive neurological test and is clinically accessible (Berciano et al 2006, Burns et al 2009, Gallardo et al 2006).

Reduced ankle joint dorsiflexion (seen at 2 years) precedes pes cavus (seen at 5 years).

The child at 3 years begins to exhibit the onset of mature gait patterns (Shepherd 1995, Tachdjian 1985, Thomson 1993), although this may range from 2 to 6 years (Payne & Isaacs 2008). The usual posture includes combination of: lumbar lordosis, knee hyperextension, genu valgum, lateral tibial torsion, symmetrical genicular position, diminished medial plantar fat pad, calcaneal eversion in weight-bearing (Cusick 1990).

From age 4–7 years the child exhibits increasing lumbar lordosis due to anterior pelvic tilting. Hip medial and lateral rotations equalize and femoral torsion reduces more slowly to approximately 25°. Maximal genu valgum resolves (Heath & Staheli 1993). Tibial torsion has reached its mature value by age 7 years; this is some 15–30° lateral. Ankle joint dorsiflexion should have range of some 10–20° and both rear and forefoot varus reduce. The eversion of the calcaneus will be reduced by 6–8 years and the forefoot plane aligns to approximate a parallel with the rear foot plane (transverse; Cusick 1990, Tachdjian 1985, Wall 2000).

Table 5.2

	Hip	Knee	Ankle
Heel strike	Flexion 45°	Flexion 0–5°	0°
Mid-stance	Flexion 15°	Flexion 20°	Flexion 10°
Toe-off	0°	Flexion 45°	Extension 20°
Swing phase	Extension reduces Flexion increases	Flexion increases Extension begins	Extension reduces Flexion (to clear ground)

The four main differences between the gait of an under 3-year-old child and that of an older child are:

1. shorter steps
2. higher cadence (rate of steps)
3. slower speed (distance/time)
4. limited single leg support.

The two main requirements to achieve a mature gait pattern are increased leg length and improved single leg/foot stability. Figure 5.13 shows the kinematic graphs of sagittal plane activity for the hip, knee and ankle. The sagittal plane is the line of progression and displays many pivotal aspects of gait biomechanics (Table 5.2).

Key Concepts

Differences in foot pressure profiles have been distinguished across three age groups: group 1: <2 years; group 2: 2–5 years; group 3: >5 years. Age-related differences in initiation patterns, force transmission and the amount of time spent on each foot segment provide evidence for maturation of children's foot pressure profiles from a flat-foot pattern in the young child to a curvilinear pattern in the older child (Alvarez et al 2008).

The attainment of a normal mature gait pattern is a gradual and complex process that depends on normal structures being adequately used. Paediatric gait evaluation is linked to knowledge of normal age expectations, developmental biomechanics, the child's environment and personality (e.g. adventurous, cautious), their developmental and family history. Neuromuscular anomalies such as cerebral palsy, muscular dystrophy or CMT need to be part of the differential diagnostic process and considered when unusual foot posture, poor gait function, gait asymmetry or gait delay are clinically evident. Liaison with medical and physical therapy colleagues is essential in such circumstances.

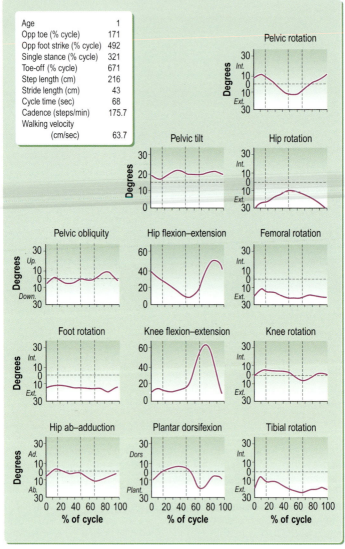

Age	1
Opp toe (% cycle)	171
Opp foot strike (% cycle)	492
Single stance (% cycle)	321
Toe-off (% cycle)	671
Step length (cm)	216
Stride length (cm)	43
Cycle time (sec)	68
Cadence (steps/min)	175.7
Walking velocity (cm/sec)	63.7

Figure 5.13 The coordination of mature gait requires integration of movements of all joints in all body planes. Observing the simultaneous kinematic activity of hip, knee and ankle is helpful is detecting the loci of gait abnormalities.

References

Alvarez C, De Vera M, Chhina H et al 2008 Normative data for the dynamic pedobarographic profiles of children. Gait and Posture 28(2):309–315

Beaty JH 1993 Knee, lower leg, foot, and ankle disorders in children. [Review] [33 refs]. Current Opinion in Pediatrics 5(3):368–373

Berciano J, Gallardo E, Garcia A et al 2006 Charcot–Marie–Tooth disease type 1A duplication with severe paresis of the proximal lower limb muscles: a long-term follow-up study. Journal of Neurology, Neurosurgery and Psychiatry 77(10):1169–1176

Burns J, Ryan MM, Ouvrier RA 2009 Evolution of foot and ankle manifestations in children with CMT1A. Muscle and Nerve 39(2):158–166

Charcot–Marie–Tooth Association Australia Inc. 2008 CMTAA brochure. http://www.cmt.org.au (accessed 19 May 2009)

Cusick BD 1990 Progressive casting and splinting for lower extremity deformities in children with neuromotor dysfunction. Therapy Skill Builders, Arizona

Cusick BD, Stuberg WA 1992 Assessment of lower-extremity alignment in the transverse plane: implications for management of children with neuromotor dysfunction. Physical Therapy 72(1):13–25

Fixsen JA, Valman HB 1981 Minor orthopaedic problems in children. British Medical Journal 283:715–717

Fuchs R, Staheli LT 1996 Sprinting and intoeing. Journal of Pediatric Orthopedics 16(4):489–491

Futagi Y, Suzuki Y, Goto M 1999 Clinical significance of plantar grasp response in infants. Pediatric Neurology 20(2):111–115

Gage JR 1993 Gait analysis: an essential tool in the treatment of cerebral palsy. Clinical Orthopaedics and Related Research 288:126–134

Gallardo E, Garcia A, Combarros O et al 2006 Charcot–Marie–Tooth disease type 1A duplication: spectrum of clinical and magnetic resonance imaging features in leg and foot muscles. Brain 129(2):426–437

Guzzetta A, Haataja L, Cowan F et al 2005 Neurological examination in healthy term infants aged 3–10 weeks. Biology of the Neonate 87(3):187–196

Heath CH, Staheli LT 1993 Normal limits of knee angle in white children – genu varum and genu valgum. Journal of Pediatric Orthopedics 13(2):259–262

Ho CS, Lin CJ, Chou YL 2000 Foot progression angle and ankle joint complex in preschool children. Clinical Biomechanics 15:271–277

Illingworth RS 1987 The development of the infant and young child: normal and abnormal, 9th edn. Churchill Livingstone, London

Payne VG, Isaacs LD 2008 Human motor development: a lifespan approach, 7th edn. McGraw-Hill, New York

Perry JP 1992 Gait analysis: normal and pathological function. Slack, Thorofare, NJ

Rose KJ, Burns J, Ryan MM et al 2008 Reliability of quantifying foot and ankle muscle strength in very young children. Muscle and Nerve 37(5):626–631

Rose SA, Ounpuu S, DeLuca PA 1991 Strategies for the assessment of pediatric gait in the clinical setting. Physical Therapy 71(12):961–980

Shepherd RB 1995 Physiotherapy in paediatrics, 3rd edn. Butterworth Heinemann, Oxford

Staheli LT 1987 Evaluation of planovalgus foot deformities with special reference to the natural history. Journal of the American Podiatric Medical Association 77(1):2–6

Sutherland DH 1978 Gait analysis in cerebral palsy. Developmental Medicine and Child Neurology 20(6):807–813

Sutherland DH 2001 The evolution of clinical gait analysis, part 1: kinesiological EMG. Gait and Posture 14:61–70

Sutherland DH 2002 The evolution of clinical gait analysis, part 2: kinematics. Gait and Posture 16:159–179

Tachdjian MO 1985 The child's foot. WB Saunders, Philadelphia

Thomson P 1993 Introduction to podopaediatrics. WB Saunders, London

Valmassy RL 1996 Clinical biomechanics of the lower extremities. Mosby, St Louis, p. 246

Zafeiriou DI 2004 Primitive reflexes and postural reactions in the neurodevelopmental examination. Pediatric Neurology 31(1):1–8

Wall EJ 2000 Practical primary pediatric orthopedics. [Review] [12 refs]. Nursing Clinics of North America 35(1):95–113

Further reading

Bruckner J 1998 The gait workbook: a practical guide to clinical gait analysis. Slack, Thorofare, NJ

Cusick BD 1990 Progressive casting and splinting for lower extremity deformities in children with neuromotor dysfunction. Therapy Skill Builders, Arizona

Payne VG, Isaacs LD 2008 Human motor development: a lifespan approach, 7th edn. McGraw-Hill, New York

Perry JP 1992 Gait analysis: normal and pathological function. Slack, Thorofare, NJ

Redmond A (forthcoming) Gait pocket book. Elsevier, Oxford

Examination of paediatric foot posture

Definition of paediatric foot posture

The anatomical position of the weight-bearing child's foot, as clinically observed in the cardinal body planes.

While the flat foot is the major concern and the more common finding, it should not be forgotten that the highly arched, supinated foot is also a concern and needs to be appreciated (see Ch. 5, Charcot–Marie–Tooth disease Key Concepts box).

Historical overview of the flat foot

The flat foot has long been regarded as a disabling problem, either immediately or potentially. The wide array of synonyms for flat feet include: pes planus (Tareco et al 1999), calcaneovalgus (Aharonson et al 1992), pes valgus (Bleck & Berzins 1977), flexible flatfoot (Wenger et al 1989), flexible pes planus Kuhn et al 1999), planovalgus (Staheli 1987), postural valgus hindfeet (Powell 1983), hypermobile flatfoot (Bordelon 1980), pronated foot (Root et al 1977).

Much has been written about flat feet, yet a precise definition remains elusive. Historically, it has been observed that people whose feet were painful were often 'flat' or observed to have a lowered medial longitudinal arch and everted (or 'valgus') heel position. Some of these people were physically limited by their flat feet and seen as 'weaker', being less able to walk or run distances or to work efficiently. From the perspective of strengthening 'weak' flat feet, various arch supports have been developed and the basic principles of these are still incorporated into orthotic therapy today.

Definition of what exactly constitutes a flat foot remains debatable, as does the premise that flat feet are problematic. There is no doubt that some flat feet are associated with pain and disability and that orthotic therapy can be beneficial (Landorf & Keenan 2000). There is, however, much doubt and dispute about children's flat feet being regarded as a problem (Bordelon 1980, 1983; Ganley 1987; Price 1982; Staheli 1987, 1999), and there is even more disagreement about the use of orthoses in children, particularly if asymptomatic (McDonald & Kidd 1998). The notion of prevention has seen children with flat feet treated with orthoses in an effort to save them from future disability. Unfortunately this notion (Bordelon 1983, Capasso 1993, D'Amico 1984, Jay & Schoenhaus 1992, Jay et al 1995, Kirby 1992, Mereday et al 1972, Valmassy 1996) is yet to be substantiated and clinicians continue to differ over the management of children with flat feet.

The definition of flat feet has not been helped by the varying techniques used to assess them. The medial longitudinal arch height, heel angle and footprints have all been used in efforts to measure the 'flatness' of feet. Clinical measures of the feet have been another area of great dissent among both clinicians and researchers. The last 20 years have seen investigation of clinical foot measures by evaluating the basic measurement principles of reliability and validity (Elveru et al 1988, Freeman 1990, Sell et al 1994). In general the reliability of these measures is poor and the validity questionable (Astrom & Arvidson 1995). Very little research has addressed the use of these measures in children's feet.

Classification of flat feet

Staheli's review articles (1987, 1994) notice the almost moralistic overtones with which the flat foot has been discussed. In contrast with the aristocratic, high-arched foot type, the flat foot was mooted as inferior. The 'low' arch was the 'fallen' arch, insinuated as being undesirable (perhaps even 'loose') as well as potentially disabling to the encumbered.

Most attempts at classifying the flat foot have focused on three aspects:

1. arch height

2. heel eversion angle

3. whether the flat foot structure is rigid or flexible.

Methods of classification have consisted of footprint assessment, X-rays and visual observation.

The arch

Great attention has been paid to the medial longitudinal arch of the foot as a way of assessing foot posture. The normal infant's foot begins as a flat foot with the medial longitudinal arch developing during childhood (Gould et al 1989, Morley 1957, Rao & Joseph 1992, Staheli 1987). It is accepted that the flatness of normal children's feet and their age are inversely proportioned (Cappello & Song 1998). The arch has been assessed using:

- footprints (Staheli 1987)
- radiographic imaging
- pedotopography (observation of the weight-bearing foot using photography; Gould et al 1989)
- clinical measurements (Gould et al 1989, Saltzman et al 1995).

Staheli (1987) devised an arch index from footprints in 441 subjects aged from 1 to 80 years. Staheli's arch index was calculated by measuring the width of the footprint arch and the width of the footprint heel and dividing the arch measure by the heel measure. Arch index results ranged broadly as 0.70–1.35 in infancy and 0.30–1.0 after childhood, indicating a decline in footprint arch width with increasing age that was surmised by the authors to be indicative of increasing arch height during childhood.

Gould's study looked specifically at the development of the child's medial longitudinal arch in subjects aged 11 months to 5 years (Gould et al 1989). The children were studied for 4 years with X-ray, clinical and pedotopographical examinations each year. This study found that medial longitudinal arch development was rapid in the first 5 years of life and was faster until 3 years of age if arch support footwear was used. It must be noted that X-ray angles were used to categorize the feet as having 'normal, slightly flat, moderate' arches, which must have been difficult when using radiographs of such young incompletely ossified feet.

Saltzman et al (1995) performed clinical and radiographic assessments in adults in an effort to validate clinical measures of the medial longitudinal arch. The best anthropometric parameter to characterize medial longitudinal arch structure was found to be a ratio of navicular height to foot length.

The heel eversion angle

Heel eversion or hindfoot valgus (Powell 1983) is generally accepted as a normal finding in young, newly walking children and is expected to reduce with age. The eversion of the heel has been repeatedly used for determining the posture of the child's foot (Wenger et al 1989). Originating in the orthopaedic literature (Morton 1937), it has been the view of podiatrists that a vertical heel (assessed by the bisection) is optimal for foot function (Fig. 6.1A, B; Root et al 1971, 1977). The basis for this principle comes from the attempts of Root (Root et al 1971, 1977) and co-authors to define all foot motion around the three cardinal body planes.

Recent research has challenged the Root model and suggested alternative methods (Dahle et al 1991; Elveru et al 1988; Keenan 1997; Menz 1995, 1998). The clinical measure of resting calcaneal stance position has guided clinicians in assessment of the child's foot posture and calcaneal eversion has been suggested (but not shown) to reduce by a degree every 12 months to a vertical position by age 7 years (Valmassy 1996). More recently a study investigating the rear foot angle in 150 children aged from 6 to 16 years (Sobel et al 1999) found that the average rear foot angle for all children was 4° valgus (ranging from 0 to 9° valgus).

Foot flexibility

The literature includes many arguments about what constitutes a flat foot versus a floppy flat foot (Luhmann et al 2000, Powell 1983), with Jack's great toe extension test seen as the delineating factor by many (Barry & Scranton 1983; Lin et al 1999; Rose et al 1985; Staheli 1987, 1999; Wenger et al 1989). Staheli (1987) has been emphatic about the distinction between pathological (rigid) and physiological (flexible) flat feet. The significance of the flexible flat foot continues to be the topic of much contention (Cohen & Cowell 1989, Garcia-Rodriguez et al 1999, Kanatli et al 2001, Lin et al 1999, Tareco et al 1999, Wenger et al 1989). The flat foot proforma (FFP) has been developed in an effort to make sense of this issue for the clinician (Evans 2007).

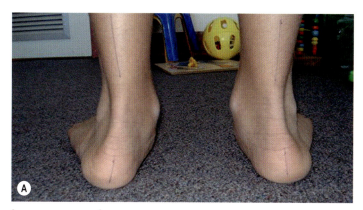

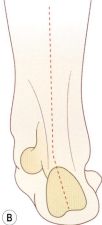

Figure 6.1 (A) The eversion angle of the heel is the main frontal/coronal plane feature of a flat foot.
(B) This reveals the associated medial drift and drop of the talus and navicular which result in a lower medial arch. Observing the medial and lateral sides of the foot for respective convexity/concavity indicates abduction of the forefoot on the rear foot. In these cases, both Jack's test and the supination resistance test require increased force, indicating a poor windlass mechanism.

Clinical Tip

Jack's test

The hallux is manually dorsiflexed while the child is standing. If the medial longitudinal arch is seen to rise, the foot is deemed a *flexible* flat foot. If the arch remains static, this test designates a *rigid* flat foot.

The rise of the medial longitudinal arch, via tightening of the plantar fascia, without muscle activity, is referred to as the *windlass mechanism,* a fundamental aspect of sagittal plane foot functioning (Aquino & Payne 2001, Cornwall & McPoil 1999a).

When applying Jack's test in adults, an immediate rising of the arch indicates greater tensile forces with the plantar fascia. In contrast, a delayed rise of the arch is associated with a more inverted heel strike, greater rear foot eversion and less re-supination (Kappel-Bargas et al 1998; Fig. 6.2).

Footprints

Footprints have been used intuitively to assess the foot's posture, the effects of orthotic intervention (Capasso 1993, Cappello & Song 1998, Sachithanandam & Joseph 1995), and especially to study flat feet in various populations (Capasso 1993, Cappello & Song 1998, Didia et al 1987, Harris & Beath 1948, Kanatli et al 2001, Lin et al 1999, Morley 1957, Rao & Jospeh 1992, Rose et al 1985, Sachithanandam & Joseph

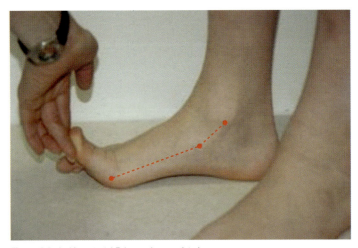

Figure 6.2 Jack's test and Feiss angle are related.

1995, Staheli 1987, Tareco et al 1999). Rose et al (1985) developed the valgus index as an early measure of flat feet. The footprint continues to be included as a proxy indicator of arch height and has formed the basis of plantar pressure measurement using:

- pedobarography (Craxford et al 1984)
- foot-ground pressure patterns (Aharonson et al 1992)
- dynamic plantar pressure systems, e.g. Emed™, Musgrave™, Vifor™ (Widhe 1997).

Whether or not footprints reflect the real morphology of the medial longitudinal arch is still controversial (Carranza-Bencano et al 1997, Volpon 1994). However, the recent development of a normative databank for foot loading patterns and foot shape parameters in new walking children does find initial correlation between dynamic pressure patterns and static footprints. This valuable and ongoing investigation has also found an increase in peak pressures of the paediatric forefoot approximating 11% per year with a simultaneous decrease of 9% per year in the midfoot area (Bosch et al 2007). Earlier, and less comprehensive, plantar pressure research found an almost three times higher load in the infant midfoot as compared to adult feet (Henning & Rosenbaum 1991). Using the Chippaux-Smirak Index in a study of 1676 children's feet, the highest percentage of lowered medial longitudinal arch was found in younger children and reduced with age, supporting the long observed physiologically increasing arch height proportional to age (Forriol & Pascual 1990, Nikalaidou & Boudolos 2006).

X-rays

Many studies have attempted to assess children's foot posture types using X-rays (Bleck & Berzins 1977, Bordelon 1980, Capasso 1993, Kanatli et al 2001, Price 1982). Staheli (1987) suggests that X-rays are only appropriate to determine the aetiology of rigid (pathological) flat feet and that these views should be taken in stance. Rose stated categorically that X-rays should be interpreted with caution when used to assess children's foot posture due to bony development and superimposition of structures (Rose et al 1985). X-rays were used to assess foot morphology in Wenger's clinical trial for foot orthoses (Wenger et al 1989) and shoes in pre-school children and also in Bordelon's uncontrolled observations (1980), hence limiting the conclusions of these studies.

Observation and the development of clinical measures

Visual appearance of the flat foot has been the basis of all other observations and has resulted in the development of quantitative measures. As previously mentioned, the arch, heel, ability of the foot to flex and form an arch and footprints have all been aspects observed and judged as constituents of the flat foot structure. X-rays have enabled an extension of visual observation, if limited to static, osseous, two-plane images. Rose was the first investigator to promote the concept of subtalar joint stability and also attempted one of the first measures of foot stability, the valgus index (Rose et al 1985). While based on the footprint, the valgus index was the first measure to focus on the rear of the heel and preceded the clinical measures developed by Root (Root et al 1977).

Podiatrists adopted the Root foot biomechanics model until the late 1980s when critical inquiry into these clinically accepted measures began (Elveru et al 1988, Mueller et al 1993, Picciano et al 1993). Developed in the 1970s, the work of Root, Orien and Weed (Root et al 1971, 1977) became the fundamental principles for podiatry students for 20 years. STJ (subtalar joint) neutral position is the essence of the Root theories, as normal feet should theoretically function from this point. It is also the reference mark from which measurements are made but lacks definition (Elveru et al 1988) as a starting point for measuring the foot (Weiner-Ogilvie et al 1997). The more recent questioning of the principles of Root biomechanics has resulted in debate and investigations into the reliability of these measures (Freeman 1990, Menz 1995, Sell et al 1994, Weiner-Ogilvie & Rome 1998, Weiner-Ogilvie et al 1997).

The reliability of traditional measures of foot posture

There are many measures of foot posture which can be used by clinicians. Overall, reliability of the traditional Root measures of foot posture has been found lacking. Some measures (e.g. navicular height) display acceptable reliability (Mathieson et al 2004, Sell et al 1994, Weiner-Ogilvie & Rome 1998) while others (e.g. resting calcaneal stance position and neutral calcaneal stance position) are less reliable. Neutral calcaneal stance position involves the locating of subtalar joint neutral position (Elveru et al 1988, Keenan 1997, Menz 1995, Pierrynowski et al 1996). The unsatisfactory reliability of neutral calcaneal stance position requires podiatrists to question the use of this measure for orthotic prescription. The validity of these measures has been very sparsely investigated (Backer & Kofoed 1989, Herbsthofer et al 1998, Schon et al 1998, Weseley et al 1969).

A number of observational assessment scales have been developed to try and address the issue of the poor reliability of foot measures. Most recently has been the development of the foot posture index (FPI; Redmond 2000; Redmond et al 2001a, 2001b), which is now used as the FPI-6 (Keenan et al 2006, Redmond et al 2006).

Foot posture index (FPI-6)

As described by Redmond (2000), the FPI-6 consists of six specific criteria:

1. talar head palpation
2. curves above and below lateral malleolus
3. inversion/eversion of the calcaneus
4. bulge in the region of the TNJ
5. congruence of medial longitudinal arch
6. abduction/adduction of the forefoot on rear foot.

Figure 6.4 and Table 6.1 illustrate the six individual FPI criteria as observed and scored. The index identifies foot types, i.e. supinated, neutral or pronated, by its scoring system (Redmond 2000, Redmond et al 2001a). The inter-rater reliability of the FPI (both the initial FPI-8 and the modified FPI-6) has been found to vary (Evans et al 2003a, Cornwall et al 2008), but is better than many other measures. The validity of the FPI has also been investigated (Keenan et al 2006, Schartfbillig et al 2004). The FPI-6 is a useful clinical tool.

Supination resistance test

A simple test used to estimate the magnitude of pronatory moments is the supination resistance test (Kirby 1992; Fig. 6.3). The foot is manually

Table 6.1					
FPI-6 criterion/ score	**−2**	**−1**	**0**	**+1**	**+2**
1. Talar head palpation	Lateral	Slight lateral	Equal	Slight medial	Medial
2. Lateral ankle curves (lower or *infra* curve)	Infra straight	Infra slight straight	Equal	Infra slight curve	Infra curved
3. Calcaneal position	Marked inversion	Slight inverted	Vertical	Slight everted	Marked eversion
4. Talonavicular joint	Marked indent	Slight indent	Flat	Slight bulge	Marked bulge
5. Medial arch	Flat arch	Lower arch	Normal arch	Moderate arch	High arch
6. Forefoot abduction/ adduction	Only medial toes seen	More medial toes	Equal medial and lateral toes	More lateral toes	Only lateral toes

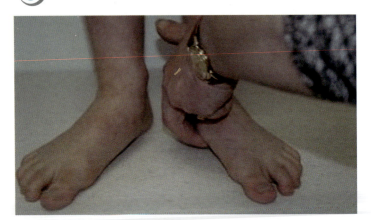

Figure 6.3 The supination resistance test.

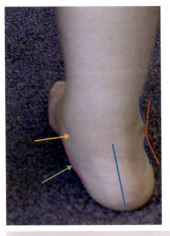

1. Talar head palpation
• Head of talus is palpated and scored for being variably from lateral to medial.

2. Lateral ankle curves
• curvatures above and below the lateral malleolus are observed and scored for curvature.

3. Inv/eversion of calcaneus
• The heel angle is observed and scored from inverted to vertical to everted.

4. Bulge of talo-navicular joint area
• The TNJ is observed and scored from flattened to bulging.

5. Medial arch congruence
• Arch is observed and scored for height and curvature.

6. Abd/adduction of forefoot on rearfoot
• Foot is observed and scored for forefoot abduction to adduction from the heel.

Figure 6.4 FPI-6 diagram illustrating the criteria 1–6 as visually observed.

supinated and the force required is assessed as being low, moderate or high. The higher the force required, the greater the supination resistance and the stronger the pronatory forces. The force needed to supinate the foot is scaled from 0 to 5. The reliability of the supination resistance test has been found to be good (ICC = 0.89) (Noakes & Payne 2003). The supination resistance test correlates moderately with mechanical loading ($r = 0.57$) and the FPI-8 ($r = 0.60$). The mean supination resistance has been assessed as 113.5 N ± 30.5 N in adult subjects (Payne et al 2003).

Similarly to STJ palpation, the supination resistance test is a useful guide for orthotic selection/prescription. In basic terms, the greater the supination resistance test, the greater the emphasis on anti-pronatory orthotic features, namely medial skive, inverted pour, medial rear foot post flare, etc.

Longitudinal arch angle (Feiss line)

The Feiss line connects the medial malleolus, the navicular and the first metatarsal head on the medial aspect of the weight-bearing foot (Fig. 6.4). In Jack's test, extension of the first metatarsophalangeal joint checks:

- foot flexibility (a rigid foot will not move)
- the onset of the windlass mechanism by tensioning the plantar fascia.

The Feiss line (malleolus – navicular – first metatarsal head) increases when Jack's test activates supination and raises the arch height. Investigation of the longitudinal arch angle found a mean value approximating 140° ± 6°, with only small associated error (SEM = 1.3°).

The reliability of the Feiss line is very good (ICC = 0.97), and there is good correlation between this angle when static and in gait ($r = 0.97$).

The angle of the Feiss line for adults is:

- 130–150°   normal foot
- <130°   pronated foot
- >150°   supinated foot (McPoil & Cornwall 2005).

Ankle range

The standing lunge test has long been known to correlate with functional ankle range and to be predicative of sporting injury. An average of 35° ankle dorsiflexion is required for normal adult gait (Bennell et al 1998). Children's ankle range assessment is generally an unreliable measure, as typically assessed when the child is non-weight-bearing (Evans & Scutter 2006). Clinically, I suggest looking at a child's ability to squat, heel walk and increase stride length (without early heel lift).

Current view of children's foot posture

From the research that has explored this area, it seems likely that the examination of young children's feet may require a different approach from adult feet (Evans 2007, Evans et al 2003a, 2003b, 2004).

> ### *Clinical* Tip
>
> The use of varying forms of in-shoe devices and orthoses in *symptomatic* children is generally supported (Evans 2003, McDonald & Kidd 1998, Mereday et al 1972, Rodgers 1999, Wenger et al 1989). In most cases a prefabricated and relatively inexpensive orthotic device will suffice. Footwear needs to be optimized for the child's circumstances primarily (Ch. 14).

The use of orthoses in adults is well supported, with positive effects on pain and foot deformity (Landorf et al 2000). There is much less evidence to support the use of any form of orthosis in children without pain (McDonald & Kidd 1998) and the notion of 'correcting' a child's foot posture by utilizing orthoses is, at best, tenuous given the quality of the research to date (Bordelon 1980, 1983; Wenger et al 1989).

Opinion is still divided about whether there is a need to intervene when the child's foot posture is 'flat' (Staheli 1999). Orthopaedists generally accept the use of orthoses in symptomatic children and podiatrists have developed a better appreciation of developmental trends of the paediatric foot and also the doubt surrounding mechanical intervention in asymptomatic children (Evans 2003, McDonald & Kidd 1998). The Cochrane Library systematic review provides the best available scientific evidence for intervention (Rome et al 2006; Table 6.2).

The flat foot proforma (FFP): a clinical pathway

Recognizing the clinical dilemma and building on clinical guidelines (Harris et al 2004), the flat foot proforma (FFP) is a recent attempt at classifying children's flat feet to help direct clinical practice (Evans 2007, 2008a) (Appendix 6.1). The FFP has been developed by the author by incorporating clinical guidelines (Harris et al 2004) with results from investigations into the reliability and validity of children's foot measures (Evans & Scutter, 2006; Evans et al 2003a, 2003b, 2003c, 2004) and the Cochrane Library review (Rome et al 2006). Recent reliability testing of the FFP has resulted in a revised version (the paediatric-FFP/p-FFP). The p-FFP has fewer items, demonstrated levels of inter-rater reliability and is quicker to use (Evans 2008b) (Appendix 6.2).

Table 6.2 Summary of the findings of the three randomized controlled trials investigating the use of foot orthoses in children with flat feet

	Wenger et al 1989	Powell et al 2005	Whitford & Esterman 2007
Number of subjects	98	40	180
Age	1–6	5–19	7–11
Condition	Flexible flat feet	Juvenile arthritis, Foot pain for 1–24 months	'Flexible excessive pronation'
Trial groups	Shoe Helfet heel cups UCBL orthoses Control	Athletic shoes Neoprene insoles Custom orthoses	Generic orthoses Custom orthoses Control
Outcome measures	X-rays	Pediatric pain questionnaire Timed walking Foot function index Ped QoL (physical)	Motor skills Physical activity Self-perception
Findings	No significant difference between groups	Orthoses group showed significant improvement in: pain, function, QoL	No significant difference between groups

Alternative clinical measures to monitor treatment efficacy

If foot orthoses are to be used, clinicians need to demonstrate their efficacy for ongoing use to be justified. Two user-friendly methods of monitoring treatment effect for an individual clinical case are the single case experimental design and the patient generated index.

1. Single case experimental design (SCED)

The SCED is a useful clinical research tool that can identify cause–effect relationships without large sample sizes. By definition this 'n = 1' design can be easily used for clinical recording about treatment efficacy for an individual case. SCED has limitations in terms of the level of evidence (Portney & Watkins 2000); it uses the principles of 'control' to establish a causal relationship. SCEDs allow conclusions to be drawn about the effects of an intervention based on the responses of a single subject under controlled conditions (Evans 2003; Table 6.3).

Table 6.3 Single case experimental design (SCED)

The essential feature of the SCED is the withdrawal of a treatment after initial clinical improvement. Without this step, intervention is presumed effective, but may have coincided with a natural resolution. Deterioration toward the baseline pain when treatment is withdrawn better tests treatment effect, justifies the treatment (pathway 1) and can avert unnecessary ongoing treatment and associated expense (pathway 2). Interventions can also be compared using an SCED design (pathway 3).

	Baseline	Treatment 1	Withdrawal	Treatment 2
Untested treatment pathway	A Pain	B No pain	–	–
SCED pathway 1	A Pain	B No pain	A Baseline pain returns	B Treatment supported
SCED pathway 2	A Pain	B No pain	A No baseline pain	– Treatment not supported
SCED pathway 3	A Pain	B Less pain	A Baseline pain returns	C No pain, treatment C better than B

Outcome measures for pain can include tools to assess pain attributes.
Pain intensity can be recorded using a visual analogue scale in older (numerate) children, or a pictorial faces scale (happy-less happy-blank-unhappy-very unhappy) in younger children (Wong-Baker faces scale; Abu-Saad & Hamers 1997, McGrath et al 2000).
Pain frequency can be recorded as the number of episodes for each SCED phase.
The frequency of using pain medication can also be recorded.

2. Patient generated index (PGI)

The PGI is a quality of life measure which addresses an individual's expectations versus experiences of clinical management outcomes. It is known that 'disease' outcome measures are often narrow and do not address satisfaction or feelings (Ruta et al 1994). There may be a use for measures which are less physical but more meaningful to the individual concerned (Carr & Higginson 2001; Table 6.4).

Clinical Tip

Utilizing the SCED and the PGI reduces the presumption that treatment, rather than natural resolve, has benefited the patient. This is very important in paediatric practice where maturation is an active process.

Table 6.4 The patient generated index (PGI)

The PGI involves the patient (in this case, the child with flat feet and their parents) specifying areas affected by the problem, e.g. poor running, leg aches after activity, shoe wear/comfort, angle of gait. The child/parents are then asked to rate each item's affect (out of 10) and then to weight the importance of each item. The index score (affects times weighted importance) reflects reality versus clinical expectations and is very useful for pre- and post-treatment comparisons (Patel et al 2003). Using this method, a broader, individualized range of affected areas are assessed at baseline and in response to treatment measures.

Area affected	Score of 10	Spend points	PGI	Tx	Score of 10	Spend points	PGI
	10	4	4.0		2	1	0.2
Extra activity	8	1	0.8		4	1	0.4
Running	3	2	0.6		1	3	0.4
Keeping up (with peers)	5	3	1.5		1	5	0.5
Panadol	Daily	0	0		0	0	0

Monitoring methodically, it is possible to identify treatments which are demonstrably efficacious, eliminating unnecessary interventions. This approach removes much of the criticism of 'over prescription' of foot orthoses in children with typical flat feet.

Prevalence

Prevalence estimates have ranged broadly, which is understandable given the variations of definition. Estimates from as low as 2.7% to 12.3% (Garcia-Rodriguez et al 1999) or more are reported. Recent prevalence research (Pfeiffer et al 2006) investigated 835 children aged from 3 to 6 years and found that flat foot was associated with children's age, gender and body weight. There was an inverse relationship between age and flat feet (3-year-olds 54%, 6-year-olds 24%) and predisposition for flat feet in males (boys 52%, girls 36%). Body weight was directly related to flat feet, encountered in 51% of overweight children, 62% of obese children and 42% of children with normal body weight.

This same study found that some 10% of children were using some form of foot support (orthotic device) and yet only 1–2% were overtly symptomatic. The authors commented that while treatment for paediatric flat foot seems to abound, it was their opinion that 'greater than 90% of the treatments were unnecessary' (Pfeiffer et al 2006). The issue of treatment of the paediatric flat foot with orthotic devices has long been the subject of contentious debate (Aharonson et al 1992, Harris et al 2004, Rome et al 2006, Staheli 1999).

Differential diagnosis

The p-FFP subdivides the paediatric flat foot on the basis of symptoms, development, in the context of possible genetic, neurological, muscular, collagen factors and heredity. This enables a comprehensive approach to clinical assessment.

Clinical Tip

The p-FFP directs the clinician to manage paediatric flat feet cases according to best available evidence, clinical guidelines and current research.

The rigid flat foot is unusual in comparison to the flexible flat foot, but often painful (Garcia-Rodriguez et al 1999, Luhmann et al 2000, Staheli 1999). Tarsal coalitions, peroneal spasm and vertical talus are the most common aetiologies. Trauma may be another aetiology. Tarsal coalitions are the most common of these factors and are discussed in Chapter 13.

Hypermobility clinically exaggerates the child's flat foot posture as either ligament laxity or low muscle tone result in less intrinsic support of the foot skeleton. Children with Down's syndrome usually display hypermobile feet and generalized reduced tone. Children with cerebral palsy may exhibit increased or reduced muscle tone in the specific distribution:

- hemiplegia: one side affected, i.e. left or right
- diplegia: both legs affected
- quadriplegia: both arms and legs affected
- triplegia: e.g. both legs and one arm
- monoplegia: one affected limb, usually an arm.

Premature or unwell babies are more likely to be hypotonic, as discussed in Chapter 1, and hence the relevance of including gestation term and Apgar score in initial history taking. Hypermobility may be usefully scaled using either the Beighton scale (van der Geissen et al 2001) or the lower limb assessment score (Ferrari et al 2005; Ch. 10).

Typical clinical picture

Classically, the child presents with a flat or pronated foot (Figs 6.1 and 6.3). The term 'pronation' is often misused with reference to the child's foot posture and needs to be defined and sensibly discussed. Pronation describes the triplane motion that crosses and incorporates the three cardinal body planes:

- sagittal (dorsiflexion)
- frontal (eversion)
- transverse (abduction).

(See Definition of terms for planes of motion and related positions, Fig. 2.7.)

By definition, pronation includes simultaneous triplanar motion and position in each plane, although the proportions will alter from foot to foot depending upon joint axial locations (Kirby 1987, 1989, 2000, 2001), joint shape and soft tissue status.

In the infant and young child we expect to see calcaneal eversion in closed kinetic chain (Sobel et al 1999, Tachdjian 1985, Valmassy 1996). This is the frontal plane portion of pronation which we observe. The amount of eversion usually reduces up to until 6–8 years of age (Sobel et al 1999, Tachdjian 1997, Wenger et al 1983; Ch. 4). There is suggestion of association between the wearing of shoes in early childhood and flat foot prevalence (Rao & Joseph 1992, Sachithanandam & Joseph 1995; Ch. 14).

The rationale for intervention in the 'excessively' pronated child's foot is controversial.

The association between pes planus and juvenile hallux valgus has been disputed in the literature (Kilmartin & Wallace 1992, McCluney & Tinley 2006), yet also supported (Kalen & Brecher 1988). The Manchester scale is a simple instrument for the assessment of hallux valgus (Garrow et al 2004, Menz & Munteanu 2005). The Manchester scale has been validated (in adults; Menz & Munteanu 2005) to show good correlation between clinical hallux valgus extent (as assessed: A, no deformity; B, mild deformity; C, moderate deformity; D, severe deformity) and the radiographic angle for intermetatarsal angle (first to second rays) and hallux abductus angle. Clinically, a Morton's foot type (short first metatarsal – patient often comment on their 'long second toe') is commonly seen with juvenile hallux valgus. Family history is often positive for this foot deformity across many generations. Management in children is frequently vexatious.

The concerns about a foot that is too flat relate not so much to the arch height itself, but to the stability of the involved joints, especially the talonavicular joint (Cornwall & McPoil 1999b, McPoil & Cornwall 1996).

In brief, the relevance of 'too much pronation' and gradually resulting foot deformity can be outlined as follows:

- Mistimed subtalar joint pronation results in harmful forces through the foot; it is unstable when it should be stable to receive forces from both ground reaction and body weight.
- Such hypermobility may cause instability of the foot skeleton, which in turn alters muscular leverage arms and eventual strength of the overpowered opposing muscles (increased with connective tissue hypermobility).
- Muscle dysfunction contributes to reduction of intrinsic foot skeletal support and continuation of forces over time, and results in deformation of the foot structure (increased with hypotonia).
- Mechanical, orthotic assistance aims to improve muscle function, gait efficiency and alleviate associated symptoms.

What constitutes 'excessive pronation' in the young foot?

Developmentally, we normally expect to see:

- Low medial longitudinal arch and calcaneal eversion with weight-bearing as direct compensation for open kinetic chain subtalar varus position. This reduces with age up until approximately 6–8 years of age (Tachdjian 1985).
- Some 10° of rear foot eversion and a flat foot appearance is usual in the normal new walking child (Ch. 4).
- More rear foot eversion and a flatter foot may be seen in children with ligament laxity, hypotonia or spasticity (Harris et al 2004).
- Most children's flat feet are flexible. A rigid flat foot is never normal and usually requires orthopaedic management (Luhmann et al 2000, Staheli 1999).

Considerations and treatment

When the child has a very flat foot, whatever the aetiology, their walking and general movement patterns are affected. Unstable feet, as the base of support, will result in considerable compensation of many body parts.

Children differ from adults

Assessment of the child's foot differs from that of the adult foot because one must be aware of age-appropriate developmental values and not merely treat children as small adults. Growth and associated musculoskeletal changes need to be appreciated, assessed and if necessary addressed.

Functional inflexibility is a common cause of sporting injuries in children and a basic factor that will contribute to compensation in children (Ch. 13).

Treatment options

Therapeutic options for the very flat child's foot may include:

1. shoe selection (see Ch. 14)
2. muscle group stretching and strengthening
3. in-shoe wedging
4. foot splints
5. night stretch splints } (see Ch. 15)
6. cast orthoses.

In children less than 6–8 years of age, the mainstays of treatment are options 1–4.

It is important to allow forefoot inversion to reduce, as part of normal development (Ch. 4). Thus a posted forefoot orthotic is largely inappropriate in this age group. An obvious exception is children who are so grossly compensated and dysfunctional that forefoot position is less important than the overall stance and gait benefits. This is not uncommon in children with cerebral palsy.

The in-shoe or 'triplane' wedge

The primary action of in-shoe wedge or splint therapy is aimed at stabilizing the rear foot and midfoot but not blocking the forefoot. Age-expected foot position, stance and gait are dynamic considerations and need to be well understood (Ch. 4). The basic action of simple in-shoe wedging is to provide a supinatory moment across the subtalar joint axis and to assist the maintenance of the talonavicular joints. The triplane wedge has been described and there are many variations on the basic version (Valmassy & Terrafranca 1986). The author's experience has modified the wedge form and the wedge placement within the shoe according to foot type and gait. STJ axis palpation is very useful and the trial use of felt wedging can assist in determining the final clinical effect (Kirby 1987, 1992, 2001; see Ch. 5).

Functional orthoses

It is appropriate to consider prescriptive cast orthoses when:

- simple, cheaper interventions are ineffective
- the child is symptomatic (Rome et al 2006)
- the child exhibits a propulsive three-phase (heel to toe) gait pattern
- the child is too heavy (Valmassy & Terrafranca 1986)

- the child is (>6–8 years) of the age when the flat foot is unlikely to reduce physiologically (Evans 2008a)
- special needs dictate therapy.

Clinical Tip

Expensive, customized foot orthoses are inadvisably used as a first-line approach. The evidence for using these devices in children is sparse. Only in symptomatic (or frankly asymmetrical) cases should foot orthoses be customized, as so often a less expensive option will suffice.

Evidence-based management

The best evidence for intervention in children with flat feet is provided by a systematic review in the Cochrane Library, summarized in Tables 6.3 and 6.4. The two randomized controlled trials pertaining to orthotic therapy in children with typical flexible flat feet found no evidence for the use of foot orthoses (generic or customized) in children who are asymptomatic (Wenger et al 1989, Whitford & Esterman 2007). In contrast, there is evidence from a third randomized controlled trial which demonstrated significant benefits for the use of customized foot orthoses in children with rheumatoid arthritis (Powell et al 2005). In the light of current evidence, the use of expensive, customized foot orthoses is definitely:

- unwarranted in children with asymptomatic flat feet
- indicated for children with rheumatoid arthritis.

The use of generic, inexpensive foot orthoses will often alleviate symptomatic flat feet in children and can be used judiciously in asymptomatic cases as clinically indicated (Evans 2007, 2008a; Harris et al 2004). Interventions should be paired with suitable outcome measures (e.g. patient generated index, single case experimental design) and monitored for effect and need.

Basic steps to managing children with flat feet

1. Be sure of the diagnosis – the p-FFP will assist.
2. Use the best evidence available for management – see Tables 6.2, 6.3, 6.5.
3. Monitor treatment outcomes (e.g. SCED, PGI).
4. Revisit differential diagnoses and seek paediatric medical or orthopaedic opinion if the clinical picture changes.

Table 6.5

The evidence for using foot orthoses in children with flat feet is only supported if they are part of a specific sub-group with juvenile arthritis or if they have foot pain. The indistinct line between the benefits of generic orthoses versus customized orthoses in children with foot pain (except in children with arthritis) needs to be appreciated, such that less expensive foot orthoses are the first-line approach.

	Evidence hierarchy	Interventions
	Systematic review	Customized foot orthoses for children with arthritis Orthoses (generic/custom) may help foot pain
	Randomized controlled trial	Customized foot orthoses for children with arthritis
	Cohort	None
	Case control	None
	Case series	In-shoe wedging Foot orthoses
	Non-rating studies	Foot orthoses

Appendix 6.1

Paediatric flat foot clinical care pathway

Child's name:

History	•Age	•Family Hx	•Associations	•Symptoms	•Trauma	•Activity	•Systems review	•Previous Tx
Findings	•Arch vs loading +/– weightbearing		•Rom	•Tender areas	•Gait barefoot shoes on limp		•Diagnostic studies X-ray CT MRI Bone scan Lab tests	

Diagnosis

A. Typical flexible flat foot +/– other factors
• Neurological, e.g. cerebral palsy, hypotonia
• Muscular, e.g. muscular dystrophies
• Genetic, e.g. Down's, Marfan's
• Collagen, e.g. Ehler's–Danlos, ligament laxity

B. Rigid flat foot
Vertical talus
Tarsel coalition
Peroneal spasm
Iatrogenic
Trauma

C. Skew foot

A. Typical flexible flat foot   1. Symptomatic*   or   Asymptomatic*

2. Non-development* (structural deformity progressing with age)	or	3. Developmental (structural deformity reducing with age)

Observe	L	R		**Assess**	L	R
medial arch height				ankle range		
heel eversion				forefoot/rear foot		
talar prominence				local tenderness		
lesions				gait–barefoot and shoes		
Also consider						
heel inversion				tibial, knee position		
windlass effect				tibial, femoral torsions vs positions		
obesity				muscle tone, ligament laxity		
os tibiale externum						
To assist clinical recording				*Best available clinical measures of structural form*		
RCSP				*Evans et al, JAPMA 93(3): 203–213, 2003*		
Navicular height				FPI-6: TNJ congruence		
Ages 4–6 FPI-6: calcaneal position				FPI-6: MLA height		
				Ages 8–14 forefoot/rear foot position		

* Basic treatment options
• Orthotics
  -generic
  -wedges
  -customized
• Stretching
Monitor: Single case design
     Patient generated index

① **Treat**
② **Monitor**
③ **Leave alone**

Plan:

Date:

Clinical pathway © Angela M. Evans PhD, 2007

To be used in conjunction with: Diagnosis & treatment of pediatric flatfoot, Harris EJ et al, J Foot & Ankle Surg 43(6): 341-370, 2004.

Appendix 6.2

Paediatric flat foot proforma (p-FFP)

Child's name: _____ Age: _____

History	•Family Hx	•Associations	•Symptoms	•Trauma	•Activity	•Systems review	•Previous Tx

Findings	•Tender areas		•Gait	•Diagnostic studies (OK/+/++)			
	• Y/N		barefoot/shoes on				
	•site/s		• ADG				
			• limp Y/N				

Diagnosis (select A/B/C)	A. Typical flexible flat foot+/– other factors	B. Rigid flat foot	C. Skew foot
	Neurological, e.g. Cerebral palsy, hypotonia	Vertical talus	Metarsus adductus
	Muscular, e.g. Muscular dystrophies	Tarsal coalition	
	Genetic, e.g. Down's, Marfan's	Peroneal spasm	
	Collagen, e.g. Ehler's–Danlos, ligament laxity	Iatrogenic	
		Trauma	

A. Typical flexible flat foot   1. Symptomatic*   or   2. Non-development*   or   3. Developmental
(Select A 1/2/3)   Asymptomatic*   (structural deformity progressing with age)   (structural deformity reducing with age)

Observe	L	R	Measure	L	R
Medial arch height (OK/reduced)			Navicular height (mm)		
Heel eversion (OK/everted)			RCSP (inverted/everted)		
Heel eversion with tip toe (Y/N)			Consider		
Tibial, knee positions (medial/OK/lateral)			Muscle tone (Y/N)		
			Ligament laxity (Y/N)		

Assessment date: _____

Action plan: (Tick)

1   **Treat**   ☐

2   **Monitor**   ☐

3   **Leave alone**   ☐

Plan: _____   Date: _____

To be used in conjunction with:
Diagnosis & treatment of pediatric flatfoot. Harris EJ et al. J Foot & Ankle Surg 43(6): 341-370, 2004.
The flat foot child – to treat or not to treat, what is the clinician to do? Evans AM, J Am Podiatr Med Assoc (Sept/Oct), 2008

p-FFP © Angela M. Evans, phD 2008

References

Abu-Saad HH, Hamers JP 1997 Decision-making and paediatric pain: a review. [Review] [40 refs]. Journal of Advanced Nursing 26(5):946–952

Aharonson Z, Arcan M, Steinback TV 1992 Foot–ground pressure pattern of flexible flatfoot in children, with and without correction of calcaneovalgus. Clinical Orthopaedics and Related Research (278):177–182

Aquino A, Payne C 2001 Function of the windlass mechanism in excessively pronated feet. Journal of the American Podiatric Medical Association 91(5):245

Astrom M, Arvidson T 1995 Alignment and joint motion in the normal foot. Journal of Sport and Physical Therapy 22(5):216–222

Backer M, Kofoed H 1989 Passive ankle mobility. Clinical measurement compared with radiography. Journal of Bone and Joint Surgery – British Volume 71:696–701

Barry RJ, Scranton PE, Jr 1983 Flat feet in children. Clinical Orthopaedics and Related Research (181):68–75

Bennell K, Talbot R, Wajsweiner H et al 1998 Intra-rater and inter-rater reliability of a weight-bearing lunge measure of ankle dorsiflexion. Australian Journal of Physiotherapy 44:175–179

Bleck EE, Berzins UJ 1977 Conservative management of pes valgus with plantar flexed talus, flexible. Clinical Orthopedics and Related Research (122):85–94

Bordelon RL 1980 Correction of hypermobile flatfoot in children by molded insert. Foot and Ankle 1(3):143–150

Bordelon RL 1983 Hypermobile flatfoot in children: comprehension, evaluation, and treatment. Clinical Orthopaedics and Related Research (181):7–14

Bosch K, Gerss J, Rosenbaum D 2007 Preliminary normative values for foot loading parameters of the developing child. Gait and Posture 26(2):238–247

Capasso G 1993 Dynamic varus heel cup: a new orthosis for treating pes planovalgus. Italian Journal of Orthopaedics and Traumatology 19(1):113–123

Cappello T, Song KM 1998 Determining treatment of flatfeet in children. [Review] [28 refs]. Current Opinion in Pediatrics 10(1):77–81

Carr AJ, Higginson IJ 2001 Are quality of life measures patient centred? BMJ 322(7298):1357–1360

Carranza-Bencano A, Zamora-Navas P, Fernandez V 1997 Viladot's operation in the treatment of the child's flatfoot. Foot and Ankle International 18(9):544–549

Cohen J, Cowell HR 1989 Corrective shoes [editorial]. Journal of Bone and Joint Surgery – American Volume 71(6):799

Cornwall MW, McPoil TG 1999a Three-dimensional movement of the foot during the stance phase of walking. Journal of the American Podiatric Medical Association 89(2):56–66

Cornwall MW, McPoil TG 1999b Relative movement of the navicular bone during normal walking. Foot and Ankle International 20(8): 507–512

Cornwall MW, McPoil TG, Lebec M et al 2008 Reliability of the modified foot posture index. Journal of the American Podiatric Medical Association 98(1):7–13

Craxford AD, Minns RJ, Park C 1984 Plantar pressures and gait parameters: a study of foot shape and limb rotations in children. Journal of Pediatric Orthopedics 4(4):477–481

Dahle LK, Mueller M, Delitto A 1991 Visual assessment of foot type and relationship of foot type to lower extremity injury. Journal of Sport and Physical Therapy 14(2):70–74

D'Amico JC 1984 Developmental flatfoot. Clinics in Podiatry 1(3): 535–546

Didia BC, Omu ET, Obuoforibo AA 1987 The use of footprint contact index II for classification of flat feet in a Nigerian population. Foot and Ankle 7(5):285–289

Elveru RA, Rothstein JM, Lamb RR 1988 Methods for taking subtalar joint measurements: a clinical report. Physical Therapy 68:678–682

Evans AM 2003 Relationship between 'growing pains' and foot posture in children: single-case experimental designs in clinical practice. Journal of the American Podiatric Medical Association 93(2):111

Evans AM 2007 The flat footed child – to treat or not to treat, what is the clinician to do? Book of Abstracts. 22nd Australasian Podiatry Conference, pp. 15–16

Evans AM 2008a The flat-footed child – to treat or not to treat, what is the clinician to do? Journal of the American Podiatric Medical Association 98(5):386–393

Evans AM 2008b The paediatric flat foot – what is the clinician to do? Society of Chiropodists and Podiatrists Annual Conference and Exhibition [Abstract]

Evans AM, Scutter S 2006 Sagittal plane range of motion of the pediatric ankle joint: a reliability study. Journal of the American Podiatric Medical Association 96(5):418–422

Evans AM, Copper AW, Scharfbillig RW et al 2003a Reliability of the foot posture index and traditional measures of foot position. Journal of the American Podiatric Medical Association 93(3):203

Evans AM, Scutter SD, Iasiello H 2003b Measuring the paediatric foot – a criterion validity and reliability study of navicular height in 4-year-old children. The Foot 13(2):76–82

Evans AM, Scutter S, Iasiello H 2003c Sonographic investigation of the paediatric navicular – an exploratory study in four year old children. Journal of Diagnostic Medical Sonography 19(4):217–221

Evans AM, Scharfbillig R, Scutter S 2004 The validity of clinical podiatric foot measures – sonographic and radiological research. Australasian Journal of Podiatric Medicine 38(1):7–11

Ferrari J, Parslow C, Lim E 2005 Joint hypermobility: the use of a new assessment tool to measure lower limb hypermobility. Clinical and Experimental Rheumatology 23(3):413–420

Forriol F, Pascual J 1990 Footprint analysis between three and seventeen years of age. Foot and Ankle 11(2):101–104

Freeman AC 1990 A study of the inter-tester and intra-tester reliability in the measurement of resting calcaneal stance position and neutral calcaneal stance position. Australian Podiatrist (June):10–13

Ganley JV 1987 Podopediatrics: the past, present, and future c hallenge. Journal of the American Podiatric Medical Association 77(8):393

Garcia-Rodriguez A, Martin-Jimenez F, Carnero-Varo M et al 1999 Flexible flat feet in children: a real problem? Pediatrics 103(6):e84

Garrow AP, Silman AJ, Macfarlane GJ 2004 The Cheshire foot pain and disability survey: a population survey assessing prevalence and associations. Pain 110:378–384

Gould N, Moreland M, Alvarez R et al 1989 Development of the child's arch. Foot and Ankle 9(5):241–245

Harris EJ, Vanore JV, Thomas JL et al 2004 Diagnosis and treatment of pediatric flatfoot. Journal of Foot and Ankle Surgery 43:341–373

Harris RI, Beath T 1948 Hypermobile flatfoot with short tendo-achilles. Journal of Bone and Joint Surgery – American Volume 30:116–138

Henning EM, Rosenbaum D 1991 Pressure distribution patterns under the feet of children in comparison with adults. Foot and Ankle 11(5):306–311

Herbsthofer B, Eckardt A, Rompe JD 1998 Significance of radiographic angle measurements in evaluation of congenital clubfoot. Archives of Orthopaedics and Trauma Surgery 117:324–328

Jay RM, Schoenhaus HD 1992 Hyperpronation control with a dynamic stabilizing innersole system. Journal of the American Podiatric Medical Association 82(3):149–153 [erratum 1995 Journal of the American Podiatric Medical Association 85(5):248]

Jay RM, Schoenhaus HD, Seymour C et al 1995 The dynamic stabilizing innersole system (DSIS): the management of hyperpronation in children. Journal of Foot and Ankle Surgery 34(2):124–131

Kalen V, Brecher A 1988 Relationship between adolescent bunions and flatfeet. Foot and Ankle 8(6):331–336

Kanatli U, Yetkin H, Cila E 2001 Footprint and radiographic analysis of the feet. Journal of Pediatric Orthopedics 21(2):225–228

Kappel-Bargas A, Woolf RD, Cornwall MW et al 1998 The windlass mechanism during normal walking and passive first metatarsalphalangeal joint extension. Clinical Biomechanics 13(3):190–194

Keenan A-M 1997 A clinician's guide to the practical implications of the recent controversy of foot function. Australasian Journal of Podiatric Medicine 31(3):87–93

Keenan A-M, Redmond AC, Horton M et al 2006 The foot posture index: Rasch analysis of a novel, foot specific outcome measure. Rheumatology 45(1):i128

Kilmartin TE, Wallace WA 1992 The significance of pes planus in juvenile hallux valgus. Foot and Ankle 13(2):53–56

Kirby KA 1987 Methods for determination of positional variations in the subtalar joint axis. Journal of the American Podiatric Medical Association 77(5):228

Kirby KA 1989 Rotational equilibrium across the subtalar joint axis. Journal of the American Podiatric Medical Association 79(1):1

Kirby KA 1992 Evaluation and non-operative management of pes valgus. In: DeValentine SJ (ed) Foot and ankle disorders in children. Churchill Livingstone, New York, pp. 307–308

Kirby KA 2000 Biomechanics of the normal and abnormal foot. Journal of the American Podiatric Medical Association 90(1):30

Kirby KA 2001 Subtalar joint axis location and rotational equilibrium theory of foot function. Journal of the American Podiatric Medical Association 91(9):465

Kuhn DR, Shibley NJ, Austin WM et al 1999 Radiographic evaluation of weight-bearing orthotics and their effect on flexible pes planus. Journal of Manipulative and Physiological Therapeutics 22(4): 221–226

Landorf KB, Keenan AM 2000 Efficacy of foot orthoses. What does the literature tell us? Journal of the American Podiatric Medical Association 90(3):149

Lin CJ, Lin SC, Huang W 1999 Physiological knock-knee in preschool children: prevalence, correlating factors, gait analysis, and clinical significance. Journal of Pediatric Orthopedics 19(5):650–654

Luhmann SJ, Rich MM, Schoenecker PL 2000 Painful idiopathic rigid flatfoot in children and adolescents. Foot and Ankle International 21(1):59–66

McCluney JG, Tinley P 2006 Radiographic measurements of patients with juvenile hallux valgus compared with age-matched controls: a cohort investigation. Journal of Foot and Ankle Surgery 45(3):161–167

McDonald M, Kidd R 1998 Mechanical intervention in children: some ethical considerations. Australasian Journal of Podiatric Medicine 32(1):7–12

McGrath PA, Speechley KN, Seifert CE et al 2000 A survey of children's acute, recurrent, and chronic pain: validation of the pain experience interview. Pain 87(1):59–73

McPoil TG, Cornwall MW 1996 Relationship between three static angles of the rearfoot and the pattern of rearfoot motion during walking. Journal of Sport and Physical Therapy 23(6):370–375

McPoil TG, Cornwall MW 2005 Longitudinal arch angle. Journal of the American Podiatric Medical Association 95(2):114–120

Mathieson I, Upton D, Prior TD 2004 Examining the validity of selected measures of foot type. Journal of the American Podiatric Medical Association 94(3):275–281

Menz HB 1995 Clinical hindfoot measurement: a critical review of the literature. The Foot 5:57–64

Menz HB 1998 Alternative techniques for the clinical assessment of foot pronation. Journal of the American Podiatric Medical Association 88(3):119

Menz HB, Munteanu SE 2005 Radiographic validation of the Manchester scale for the classification of hallux valgus deformity. Rheumatology 44:1061–1066

Mereday C, Dolan CM, Lusskin R 1972 Evaluation of the University of California Biomechanics Laboratory shoe insert in 'flexible' pes planus. Clinical Orthopaedics and Related Research 82:45–58

Morley AM 1957 Knock-knee in children. BMJ 11:978–979

Morton DJ 1937 Physiological considerations in the treatment of flatfoot. Journal of Bone and Joint Surgery – British Volume 19:1052–1056

Mueller MJ, Host JV, Norton BJ 1993 Navicular drop as a composite measure of excessive pronation. Journal of the American Podiatric Medical Association 83(4):198–202

Nikalaidou ME, Boudolos KD 2006 A foot-print approach for the rational classification of foot types in young children. The Foot 16:82–90

Noakes H, Payne C 2003 The reliability of the manual supination resistance test. Journal of the American Podiatric Medical Association 93(3):185

Patel KK, Veenstra DL, Patrick DL 2003 A review of selected patient-generated outcome measures and their application in clinical trials. Value in Health 6(5):595–603

Payne C, Oates M, Noakes H 2003 Static stance response to different types of foot orthoses. Journal of the American Podiatric Medical Association 93(6):492–498

Pfeiffer M, Kotz R, Ledl T et al 2006 Prevalence of flat foot in preschool-aged children. Pediatrics 118(2):634–639

Picciano AM, Rowlands MS, Worrell T 1993 Reliability of open and closed kinetic chain subtalar joint neutral positions and navicular drop test. Journal of Sport and Physical Therapy 18(4):553–558

Pierrynowski MR, Smith SB, Mlynarczyk JH 1996 Proficiency of foot care specialists to place the rearfoot at subtalar neutral. Journal of the American Podiatric Medical Association 86(5):217–223

Portney LG, Watkins MP 2000 Foundations of clinical research: applications to practice, 2nd edn. Prentice Hall Health, Upper Saddle River, NJ

Powell HD 1983 Pes planovalgus in children. Clinical Orthopaedics and Related Research (177):133–139

Powell M, Seid M, Szer IS 2005 Efficacy of custom foot orthoses in improving pain and functional status in children with juvenile idiopathic arthriris: a randomized trial. Journal of Rheumatology 32(5):943–950

Price CT 1982 Shoes don't 'cure' flatfeet. Journal of the Florida Medical Association 69(10):853–857

Rao UB, Joseph B 1992 The influence of footwear on the prevalence of flat foot: a survey of 2300 children [see comments]. Journal of Bone and Joint Surgery – British Volume 74(4):525–527

Redmond AC 2000 The Foot Posture Index. [Unpublished]

Redmond AC, Burns J, Crosbie J et al 2001a An initial appraisal of the validity of a criterion based, observational clinical rating system for foot posture. Journal of Sport and Physical Therapy 31(3):160 [Abstract]

Redmond AC, Crosbie J, Peat J et al 2001b A new criterion based, composite clinical rating system for the quantification of foot posture: its validation and use in clinical trials. Book of Abstracts, pp. 55–57. [Abstract]

Redmond AC, Crosbie J, Ouvrier R 2006 Development and validation of a novel rating system for scoring foot posture: the foot posture index. Clinical Biomechanics 21(1):89–98

Rodgers E 1999 Growing pains [Letter; Comment]. Australian Family Physician 28(5):428

Rome K, Ashford RL, Evans AM 2006 Non-surgical interventions for paediatric pes planus. Cochrane Database of Systematic Reviews (4):1–7

Root ML, Orien WP, Weed JH et al 1971 Biomechanical examination of the foot. Clinical Biomechanics Corporation, Los Angeles

Root ML, Weed JH, Orien WP 1977 Normal and abnormal function of the foot. Clinical Biomechanics Corporation, Los Angeles

Rose GK, Welton EA, Marshall T 1985 The diagnosis of flat foot in the child. Journal of Bone and Joint Surgery – British Volume 67(1):71–78

Ruta DA, Garratt AM, Leng M et al 1994 A new approach to the measurement of quality of life: the patient-generated index. Medical Care 32:1109–1126

Sachithanandam V, Joseph B 1995 The influence of footwear on the prevalence of flat foot: a survey of 1846 skeletally mature persons. Journal of Bone and Joint Surgery – British Volume 77(2):254–257

Saltzman CL, Nawoczenski DA, Talbot KD 1995 Measurement of the medial longitudinal arch. Archives of Physical Medicine and Rehabilitation 76:45–49

Scharfbillig R, Evans AM, Copper AW et al 2004 Criterion validation of four criteria of the foot posture index. Journal of the American Podiatric Medical Association 94(1):31–38

Schon LC, Weinfeld SB, Horton GA 1998 Radiographic and clinical classification of acquired midtarsus deformities. Foot and Ankle International 19:394–398

Sell KE, Verity TM, Worrell TW et al 1994 Two measurement techniques for assessing subtalar joint position: a reliability study. Journal of Sport and Physical Therapy 19(3):162–167

Sobel E, Levitz S, Caselli M et al 1999 Natural history of the rearfoot angle: preliminary values in 150 children. Foot and Ankle International 20(2):119–125

Staheli LT 1987 Evaluation of planovalgus foot deformities with special reference to the natural history. Journal of the American Podiatric Medical Association 7(1):2–6

Staheli LT 1994 Footwear for children. [Review] [50 refs]. Instructional Course Lectures 43:193–197

Staheli LT 1999 Planovalgus foot deformity. Current status [see comments]. [Review] [28 refs]. Journal of the American Podiatric Medical Association 89(2):94–99

Tachdjian MO 1985 The child's foot. WB Saunders, Philadelphia

Tachdjian MO 1997 Clinical pediatric orthopedics. Appleton & Lange, Stamford, CT

Tareco JM, Miller NH, MacWilliams BA et al 1999 Defining flatfoot. Foot and Ankle International 20(7):456–460

Valmassy RL 1996 Clinical biomechanics of the lower extremities. Mosby, St Louis, p. 246

Valmassy RL, Terrafranca N 1986 The triplane wedge. Journal of the American Podiatric Medical Association 76(12):672–675

van der Geissen LJ, Liekens D, Rutgers KJ et al 2001 Validation of Beighton score and prevalence of connective tissue signs in 773 Dutch children. Journal of Rheumatology 28(12):2726–2730

Volpon JB 1994 Footprint analysis during the growth period. Journal of Pediatric Orthopedics 14:83–85

Weiner-Ogilvie S, Rome K 1998 The reliability of three techniques for measuring foot position. Journal of the American Podiatric Medical Association 88(8):381–386

Weiner-Ogilvie S, Rendall GC, Abboud RJ 1997 Reliability of open kinetic chain subtalar joint measurement. The Foot 7:128–134

Wenger DR, Mauldin D, Morgan D et al 1983 Foot growth rate in children age one to six years. Foot and Ankle 3(4):207–210

Wenger DR, Mauldin D, Speck G 1989 Corrective shoes and inserts as treatment for flexible flatfoot in infants and children [see comments]. Journal of Bone and Joint Surgery – American Volume 71(6):800–810

Weseley MS, Koval R, Kleiger B 1969 Roentgen measurement of ankle flexion–extension motion. Clinical Orthopaedics and Related Research 65:167–172

Whitford D, Esterman A 2007 A randomized controlled trial of two types of in-shoe orthoses in children with flexible excess pronation of the feet. Foot and Ankle International 28(6):715–723

Widhe T 1997 Foot deformities at birth: a longitudinal prospective study over a 16-year period. Journal of Pediatric Orthopedics 17(1):20–24

Further reading

DeValentine SJ 1992 Foot and ankle disorders in children. Churchill Livingstone, New York

Thomson P 1993 Introduction to podopaediatrics. WB Saunders, London

Valmassy RL 1996 Clinical biomechanics of the lower extremities. Mosby, St Louis

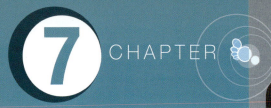

7

CHAPTER

Growing pains

Definition of growing pains

Non-specific leg pain which affects otherwise healthy children. Defined by exclusion, the inclusion criteria for growing pains are: intermittent pains in the muscles (not the joints) of both legs, which occur at night-time.

Introduction

Growing pains were first described as a distinct clinical entity by the French physician Marcel Duchamp in 1823 (Abu-Arafeh 1996). Since that time, the condition has occupied both the medical literature and the consultations of various health professionals with convincing frequency (Macarthur et al 1996). The term 'growing pains', as enigmatic as it is accessible (Brown et al 1998), has been disputed by some (Manners 1999) and challenged by others (Al-Khattat & Campbell 2000), yet remains part of everyday language (Welch 2004).

Diagnosis

One of the difficulties with growing pains is the lack of definition. There is no single pathognomonic test for growing pains so it continues to be a diagnosis of exclusion (Peterson 1977, 1986), as shown in Table 7.1. The condition seems to affect children of all ages.

Table 7.1 Definition of growing pains: inclusion and exclusion criteria

	Inclusions	Exclusions
Nature of pain	Intermittent Some pain-free days and nights	Persistent Increasing intensity
Unilateral or bilateral	Bilateral	Unilateral
Location of pain	Anterior thigh, calf, posterior knee – in muscles	Joint pain
Onset of pain	Late afternoon or evening	Pain still present next morning
Physical examination	Normal	Swelling, erythema, tenderness Local trauma or infection Reduced joint range Limping
Laboratory tests	Normal	Objective findings, e.g. ESR, X-ray, bone scan

Aetiology

The aetiology of growing pains remains uncertain, with three main theories held. The anatomical theory (Naish & Apley 1951) suggested that orthopaedic factors such as flat feet or knock knees create increased leg muscle work. The fatigue theory (Bennie 1894) alluded to an overuse response of the leg muscles in active children. The psychological or emotional theory (Oberklaid et al 1997) has viewed growing pains in a wider pain sphere including abdominal pains and headaches (Mikkelsson et al 1997a, 1998).

There have also been preliminary links between foot posture and growing pains (Evans 2003, Naish & Apley 1951) which have subsequently been well investigated and refuted (Evans & Scutter 2007). Suggested associations of functional health with growing pains (Atar et al 1992) revealed that children with growing pains were heavier than their unaffected peers (Evans et al 2006), which may have implications for childhood obesity.

Recent studies (Hashkes et al 2004, Friedland et al 2005, Noonan et al 2004) and a review (Uziel & Hashkes 2007) have identified issues such as lowered pain thresholds (Hashkes et al 2004) in children affected by growing pains, suggesting that growing pains is a more generalized pain syndrome. Bone strength has been reported to be decreased in children with growing pains (Friedland et al 2005), especially in the tibiae, which may suggest bone fatigue as a factor. Vascular changes have been cited, but as yet not implicated, in children with growing pains (Uziel & Hashkes 2007). However, a higher occurrence of growing pains has been found in children who also experience migraine headaches (Aromaa et al 2000, Oster 1972, Mikkelsson et al 1997b).

A family pattern and tendency towards growing pains has been demonstrated, with approximately 70% of children with growing pains having an affected parent or sibling (Evans et al 2006). While many studies have implicated family patterns and responses to pain as being a part of the growing pains picture (Apley 1976, Naish & Apley 1951, Oberklaid et al 1997), there has been only preliminary investigation of effects on children's quality of life (Uziel & Hashkes 2007). There is concern that children whose pain is inadequately addressed and relieved may become adolescents and adults who cope less ably with pain, which has large social and health cost implications (Eccleston & Malleson 2003, Uziel & Hashkes 2007). It is therefore important that a frequent and prevalent childhood complaint such as growing pains be well identified and managed.

Prevalence

There are some 10 prevalence studies with estimates ranging from approximately 2% to 49% (Evans & Scutter 2004a, Williams 1928). However, many of these studies were methodologically problematic using inconsistent criteria for growing pains and investigating very different age groups and sample sizes of children. Recently the prevalence of growing pains was established as 36.9% (95% CI 32.7–41.1%) in a rigorous study of 1445 children aged 4–6 years (Evans & Scutter 2004a). This study utilized the specifically designed University of South Australia Growing Pains Questionnaire (USAGPQ), which is a useful instrument for both the clinician and the researcher (Evans & Scutter 2004b, 2004c; see Appendix 7.1).

Differential diagnosis

The clinician must always keep in mind other possible, if infrequently occurring, causes of leg pain in children. Often children undergo extensive laboratory examinations to eliminate concerns of more sinister entities (Macarthur et al 1996). Juvenile arthritis should be considered if the pains are articular in nature or associated with any clinical findings such as joint swelling or morning stiffness. A bone tumour should be considered if the pain is focal and unilateral and not only occurring at night-time. Restless

Table 7.2 Differential diagnoses for children's leg pain

Differential diagnostic considerations	Be suspicious if:	Further investigation
Juvenile arthritis	Articular, unilateral or bilateral, morning stiffness	Refer to paediatrician Blood tests
Bone tumour	Unilateral	Refer to paediatrician Bone scan
Muscle metabolism disorder	Only after increased activity, bilateral and upper limbs too	Refer to paediatrician
Fibromyalgia	Tender areas palpable	Refer to paediatrician
Restless legs	Positive family history	Refer to paediatrician
Other	If growing pains criteria in Table 7.1 are not met	Refer to paediatrician

legs (sometimes termed Ekbom's syndrome) may also be implicated or coexist (Ekbom 1975, Rajaram et al 2004). The diagnosis of growing pains is greatly assisted if the definition as depicted in Table 7.1 is adhered to. However, if the signs or symptoms are atypical the diagnosis of growing pains should not be made until other investigations rule out other possible causes. Table 7.2 outlines the differential diagnoses which should be considered if the criteria in Table 7.1 are not met. Referral to a paediatrician or to other medical personnel should be arranged if the diagnosis of growing pains does not fit, or changes from, the typical clinical picture.

Typical clinical picture

Classically the child presents with the following story from their parents: their otherwise well child has been complaining of sore, aching legs at bed-time and/or waking up in the middle of the night complaining of the same thing. The level of reported distress will vary from complaining to screaming, with crying being a fair delineator in terms of the intensity of pain. Milder presentations report the child complaining and whining and often able to be alleviated with parental reassurance, a parent rubbing the child's legs, use of a hot water bottle (or equivalent) and perhaps paracetamol. Medication is usually given when the child is very distressed and some parents report that this is the only way to settle their child, while others find non-medication measures adequate. The typical pattern of growing pain episodes is that these occur in spates, e.g. a few nights over a week and then none for perhaps a month. Most affected children experience pains between 1 and 3 monthly intervals. Some parents notice a pattern of episodes on the nights that their child has been particularly active physically and begin to predict these events. There is usually a family history of growing pains and most parents do not consult a health professional. It is probable that it is in more severe, unrelenting cases or cases without a family history that a professional is consulted.

Clinical Tip

When taking the case history of children with growing pains, it is clearly vital that the clinician is well familiar with the inclusion/exclusion criteria and appreciative of the concerns raised. The history is usually defining, but differential factors must be checked off as part of completing the examination as thoroughly as is possible for a condition with no concrete criteria. Tables 7.1 and 7.2 will greatly assist the clinician's consultation.

Unfortunately, some parents who consult a health professional can be/feel somewhat dismissed and not taken seriously. This is a pity, as growing pains is a common childhood complaint which needs to be recognized, appreciated and managed effectively as outlined below. The ill-founded view that 'there's no such thing as growing pains' needs to be dispensed with as it is both ignorant and unhelpful to parents and affected children.

Evidence-based management

There is a veritable plethora of cited ways to treat children with growing pains. Everything from heat packs, stretching, massage, paracetamol, vitamin C, magnesium and zinc supplements, stabilizing leather pelvic belts, foot orthoses and probably other options have been expounded and recommended.

Clinical Tip

The only methods which have scientific backing are muscle stretches (Baxter & Dulberg 1988) and in-shoe foot wedges/orthoses (Evans 2003).

Table 7.3 illustrates the cited interventions and their respective positioning on the evidence hierarchy model. Clearly the best evidence and thus the first-line approach for management of growing pains is a muscle stretching regime (Evans 2008). A systematic, evidence directed approach

Table 7.3 The hierarchy of evidence for the management of growing pains in children

Evidence hierarchy	Interventions
Systematic review	None
Randomized controlled trial	Muscle stretching
Cohort	None
Case control	None
Case series	In-shoe wedging
Non-rating studies	Heat Massage Paracetamol Vitamin C Mg, Zn supplements Leather belt

Table 7.4 Summary of the only randomized controlled trial (RCT) for treatment of growing pains (GP) (Baxter & Dulberg 1988)

Number of pain episodes per month	Group 1 – treatment Muscle stretching programme* ($n = 18$)	Group 2 – control Reassurance, leg rubs, acetyl salicylic acid ($n = 16$)
Beginning of trial	10	10
3 months	1	6
9 months	0	3
18 months	0	2

The RCT for management of GP revealed a statistically significant difference between the treatment and control groups of children (aged 5–14 years). However, the study was biased, with no examiner blinding. Additionally, sample sizes were small and statistical power was not calculated.
*Parents were taught a muscle stretching programme for quadriceps, hamstrings and gastroc-soleal groups. All stretches were performed twice daily (morning and evening) for 10 minutes each time.

to managing children with growing pains is outlined in the algorithm shown as Figure 7.1. Table 7.4 explicates the findings of the available clinical trial.

Remember the basic steps to managing children with growing pains are:

1. Be sure of the diagnosis – Tables 7.1 and 7.2 will assist.
2. Use the best evidence available for management – see Figure 7.1, Table 7.4.

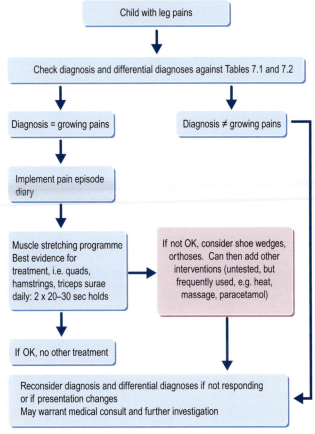

Figure 7.1 Algorithm for the diagnosis and management of children with growing pains.

3. Monitor treatment outcomes – ask parents to record pain episode frequency.
4. Revisit differential diagnoses and seek medical investigations if clinical picture changes from growing pains definition.

Appendix 7.1

Questionnaire for Parents

Thank you for answering this brief questionnaire about children's leg aches (sometimes called "growing pains"). Your response can help toward better management of this distressing condition for young children.

1. Please tick a box to answer:
    Has your child ever experienced aching legs (sometimes called "growing pains")?
    Yes?   ☐
    No?   ☐
    Don't know?   ☐

If the answer to question 1 was 'yes' please go to question 2.
If the answer to question 1 was 'no' or 'don't know please skip to question 9.

2. Please tick the box(es) which describe your child's experience of leg aches:
    (you can tick more than one box)

    Leg aches occur at night time   ☐
    Child wakes from sleep   ☐
    Child is crying   ☐
    Pain is in both legs   ☐
    Child is otherwise well   ☐

3. Please tick one box that indicates how often your child has experienced aching legs:

    Daily   ☐
    Weekly   ☐
    Monthly   ☐
    3–monthly   ☐
    6–monthly   ☐
    Other – please specify below: _____

4. Please tick the box(es) which indicate any treatments or investigations that have been given to your child: (you can tick more than one box)

    None   ☐
    Pain medication   ☐
    Foot orthotics   ☐
    X-ray   ☐
    Bone scan   ☐
    Blood test   ☐
    Other – please specify below: _____

Continued

5. Please tick a box to answer:
    Has any member of your child's family also experienced "growing pains"?

    Yes ☐
    No ☐

    Please describe the relationship of this person to your child (e.g. mother, brother, etc.): _____

6. Please tick the box(es) to answer: (you can tick more than one box)
    When your child has experienced aching leg, what have you done?

    Rubbed their legs ☐
    Hot water bottle (or similar) ☐
    Panadol ☐
    Other – please specify below: _____

7. Please tick the box(es) to answer:
    Have your child's leg pains been associated with any of the following:

    After sport ☐
    Increased activity ☐
    Rapid growth ☐
    Not wearing shoes ☐
    Flat feet ☐
    Other – please specify below: _____

8. Please circle the term which best indicates your response to the statement below:
    My child's quality of life has been reduced because of their leg aches.

    strongly agree ☐   agree ☐   uncertain ☐   disagree ☐   strongly disagree ☐

    Please specify below if you wish: _____

    Thanks! *This is the last bit*

    The following information will help me to sort children into similar groups and give clearer results from this questionnaire.

9. Could you please complete the following by circling the correct item:
    Your child's age: 4 years   5 years   6 years
    Your child's sex: male   female

    Your child's activity level: (please circle one answer below)
    very active   active   average activity   quite inactive   very inactive

Continued

10. During the last week, how happy has your child been with:
    (circle one response on each line)

	Very happy	Somewhat happy	Not sure	Somewhat unhappy	Very unhappy	Child is too young
a. How he /she looks?	1	2	3	4	5	6
b. His/her body?	1	2	3	4	5	6
c. What clothes or shoes he/she can wear?	1	2	3	4	5	6
d. His/her ability to do the same things that his/her friends do?	1	2	3	4	5	6
e. His/her health in general?	1	2	3	4	5	6

11. During the **last week**, how much of the time: (Circle one response)

	Most the time	Some of the time	A little of the time	None of the time
Did pain or discomfort interfere with your child's activities?	1	2	3	4

12. How much pain has your child had during the last week? (circle one response)

1 None   2 Very mild   3 Mild   4 Moderate   5 Severe   6 Very severe

13. During the last week, how much did pain interfere with your child's normal activities (including at home, outside of the home, and at school?) (circle one response)

1 Not at all   2 A little bit   3 Moderately   4 Quite a bit   5 Extremely

Thank you very much for completing this questionnaire and helping me with my study – I really appreciate your time. *Please return this questionnaire with the consent form in the reply paid envelope provided.*

Thank you!
Angela Evans – University of South Australia

References

Abu-Arafeh I RG 1996 Recurrent limb pain in school children. Archives of Disease in Childhood 74:336–339

Al-Khattat A, Campbell J 2000 Recurrent limb pain in childhood ('growing pains'). The Foot 10:117–123

Apley J 1976 Limb pains with no organic disease. Clinics in Rheumatic Diseases 2:487–491

Aromaa M, Sillanpaa M, Rautava P et al 2000 Pain experience of children with headache and their families: a controlled study. Pediatrics 106(2/1):270–275

Atar D, Lehman WB, Grant AD 1992 Growing pains. Physician Assistant 16(11):67–69, 90–92 [16 refs]

Baxter MP, Dulberg C 1988 Growing pains in childhood – a proposal for treatment. Journal of Pediatric Orthopedics 8(4):402–406

Bennie PB 1894 Growing pains. Archives of Pediatrics 11(5):337–347

Brown JL, Lehman WB, Peterson HA 1998 Understanding the nature of growing pains. Patient Care 32(7):63–64; 67–8; 70–71 passim [5 refs, 3 bib]

Eccleston C, Malleson P 2003 Managing chronic pain in children and adolescents. BMJ 326(7404):1408

Ekbom K 1975 Growing pains and restless legs. Acta Paediatrica Scandinavica 64:264–266

Evans AM 2003 Relationship between 'growing pains' and foot posture in children: single-case experimental designs in clinical practice. Journal of the American Podiatric Medicine Association 93(2):111

Evans AM 2008 Growing pains: contemporary knowledge and recommended practice. Journal of Foot and Ankle Research 1(1):4

Evans A, Scutter S 2004a The prevalence of 'growing pains' in young children. Journal of Pediatrics 145(2):255–258

Evans AM, Scutter SD 2004b Development of a questionnaire for parental rating of leg pain in young children: internal validity and reliability testing following triangulation. The Foot 14:42–48

Evans AM, Scutter SD 2004c A South Australian study of the prevalence of 'growing pains' in children aged four to six years. Australasian Epidemiologist 11(2):23–25

Evans AM, Scutter S 2007 Are foot posture and functional health different in children with growing pains? International Journal of Pediatrics 49(6):991–996

Evans AM, Scutter S, Lang LMG 2006 'Growing pains' in young children: a study of the profile, experiences and quality of life issues of four to six year old children with recurrent leg pain. The Foot 16(3):120–124

Friedland O, Hashkes PJ, Jaber L et al 2005 Decreased bone speed of sound in children with growing pains measured by quantitative ultrasound. Journal of Rheumatology 32(7):1354–1357

Hashkes PJ, Friedland O, Jaber L 2004 Decreased pain threshold in children with growing pains. Journal of Rheumatology 31(3):610–613

Macarthur C, Wright JG, Srivastava R 1996 Variability in physicians' reported ordering and perceived reassurance value of diagnostic tests in children with 'growing pains'. Archives of Pediatrics and Adolescent Medicine 150(10):1072–1076

Manners P 1999 Are growing pains a myth? [see comments]. [Review] [4 refs]. Australian Family Physician 28(2):124–127

Mikkelsson M, Salminen JJ, Kautiainen H 1997a Non-specific musculoskeletal pain in preadolescents: prevalence and 1-year persistence. Pain 73(1):29–35

Mikkelsson M, Sourander A, Piha J et al 1997b Psychiatric symptoms in preadolescents with musculoskeletal pain and fibromyalgia. Pediatrics 100(2/1):220–227

Mikkelsson M, Salminen JJ, Sourander A 1998 Contributing factors to the persistence of musculoskeletal pain in preadolescents: a prospective 1-year follow-up study. Pain 77(1):67–72

Naish JM, Apley J 1951 'Growing pains': a clinical study of non-arthritic limb pains in children. Archives of Disease in Childhood 26:134–140

Noonan KJ, Leiferman EM, Lampl M et al 2004 Growing pains: are they due to increased growth during recumbency as documented in a Lamb model? Journal of Pediatric Orthopedics 24(6):726–731

Oberklaid F, Amos D, Liu C et al 1997 'Growing pains': clinical and behavioral correlates in a community sample [see comments]. Journal of Developmental and Behavioral Pediatrics 18(2):102–106

Oster J 1972 Recurrent abdominal pain, headache and limb pains in children and adolescents. Pediatrics 50(3):429–436

Peterson H 1986 Growing pains. Pediatric Clinics of North America 33(6):1365–1372

Peterson HA 1977 Leg aches. Pediatric Clinics of North America 24(4):731–736

Rajaram S-S, Walters AS, England SJ 2004 Some children with growing pains may actually have restless legs syndrome. Sleep 27(4):767–773

Uziel Y, Hashkes PJ 2007 Growing pains in children. Pediatric Rheumatology Online Journal 5:5

Welch TR 2004 'Growing pains' [editorial]. Journal of Pediatrics 145(2):1A

Williams MF 1928 Rheumatic conditions in school children. The Lancet 1928:720–721

Further reading

Evans AM 2005 An investigation of leg pain ('growing pains') in children aged four to six years. Unpublished doctoral thesis, School of Health Sciences, University of South Australia, Adelaide. Online: http://arrow. unisa.edu.au:8081/1959.8/25034 Available at: http://www.library.unisa. edu.au/adt-root/public/adt-SUSA-07112005-114434/index.html (accessed 14 May 2009)

Clubfoot: talipes equinovarus

Introduction

This chapter provides a basic overview and is to be read in conjunction with the following reference sources:

1. Ponseti IV, Morcuende JA, Mosca V et al 2009 Clubfoot: Ponseti management, 3rd edn. Global HELP Organization publication (www.global-help.org). Available online as PDF file: http://www.global-help.org/publications/books/help_cfponseti.pdf (accessed 15 May 2009).

2. Evans AM, Do Van Thanh 2009 A review of the Ponseti method and development of an infant clubfoot program in Vietnam. Journal of the American Podiatric Medical Association 99(4):306–316.

The presentation of a typical clubfoot in a newborn infant is often anticipated in developed countries where prenatal screening has detected and explored this developmental aberration. Treatment is expected and while the foot will not be perfect, the child will be carefully assessed and managed assiduously by physiotherapists and orthopaedists to ensure a good outcome. The child will be expected and able to play sports in most cases.

In a developing country, the neonatal clubfoot presentation can signal a bleak future of serious disability and potential poverty for the child and their family. Hindered mobility reduces education and employment prospects. Socially the child may grow into a marginalized and impoverished adult who will depend on family support or external aid sources to survive (Gupta et al 2006, Ponseti et al 2003, Tindall et al 2005). The frequent presence of many neglected adult clubfoot deformities in many of the developing countries reinforces this reality.

The clubfoot or *talipes equinovarus* deformity has long been recognized as a serious pediatric orthopaedic problem responsible for much suffering, multiple medical interventions and often disabling outcomes for the child (Ponseti et al 2003, Tindall et al 2005, Agrawal & Pandey 2007).

The incidence of infant clubfoot varies according to ethnicity (Pandey & Pandey 2003, Tachdjian 1985). The lowest incidence is found in Chinese infants (0.39 : 1000 births) and the highest incidence found in Polynesia (6.81 : 1000 births). The incidence among Caucasian infants is approximately 1.12 : 1000 births.

Surgical correction (once thought to be the optimal management approach) has now been replaced by non-operative correction as the almost universally accepted standard of initial treatment of congenital idiopathic clubfoot (Dobbs et al 2004, Morcuende et al 2004). While there are many methods of non-operative correction (manipulation and serial casting, physical therapy and continuous passive motion), which can be successful when correctly instituted, clinical reports have found success rates of only 15–50% (Dobbs et al 2004). The frequently reported exception is the Ponseti method which has reported impressive results in both the short and long term approximating greater than 90% (Changulani et al 2006, Herzenberg et al 2002, Morcuende et al 2004, Ponseti et al 2003).

The Ponseti method has gained increasing favour globally in the last three decades, although it has been used by the original author (Dr Ignacio Ponseti) since the 1940s. The follow-up results over 35 years are very good in terms of pain and function (Cooper & Dietz 1995). In contrast, the follow-up results for primary surgical correction involving extensive soft tissue release (the Turco procedure) are not good, with long-term results showing poorly functional, painful and arthritic feet (Dobbs et al 2006). The Ponseti technique has been refined over many years and current research continues to inform our practice and method (Dobbs et al 2004, Dyer & De Vaus 2006, Haft et al 2007, Herzenberg et al 2002, Lehman et al 2003, Pirani et al 2001, Shack & Eastwood 2007).

Basic pathology

The congenital idiopathic clubfoot deformity is identified by the presence of a retracted and inverted heel (equinus), usually a medial crease on the plantar aspect of the adducted forefoot and longitudinal arch cavus. Pathognomonic to this deformity is the inability to be able to bring the foot to a plantigrade position. In unilateral cases, the clubfoot is comparatively stiff, smaller with leg muscle atrophy and shortening also common.

In terms of aetiology, a normally developing foot deforms at approximately the 16th fetal week to become a clubfoot. While genetics and environmental influences are both probable contributors, it is curious to note that a more precise mechanism(s) of aetiology is still unknown. The primary deformity centres on the shape and position of the talus and the related misplacement of the navicular.

The Ponseti method focuses on stabilizing the talus and reducing the clubfoot deformity by abducting the inverted forefoot. This allows for the calcaneus to abduct, which, in turn, allows for the ankle to be dorsiflexed (often necessitating lengthening of the Achilles tendon) (Pandey & Pandey 2003; Ponseti 1997; Ponseti et al 2003, 2006).

Types

There are three main types of clubfoot to consider when diagnosing the infant clubfoot:

1. Congenital idiopathic clubfoot: a difficult deformity that affects otherwise healthy children.
2. Resistant clubfoot: often associated with syndromes such as arthrogryposis and stiffer in nature.
3. Atypical or complex clubfoot: a short, fat, stiff clubfoot which requires a very adapted casting approach (Ponseti et al 2006).

The Ponseti method

Key Concepts

The Ponseti method is not quick, but gives the best long-term results for the life of the growing child.

From the time of initial assessment and discussion with parents, the following process is followed:

1. Assess the clubfoot type.
2. Score the severity using the Pirani score (Fig. 8.1).
   a. Assesses initial clubfoot severity.
   b. Shown to be a reliable tool (Evans 2007).
   c. Predicts the need for Achilles tenotomy (Shack & Eastwood 2007) and is prognostic (Dyer & De Vaus 2006).

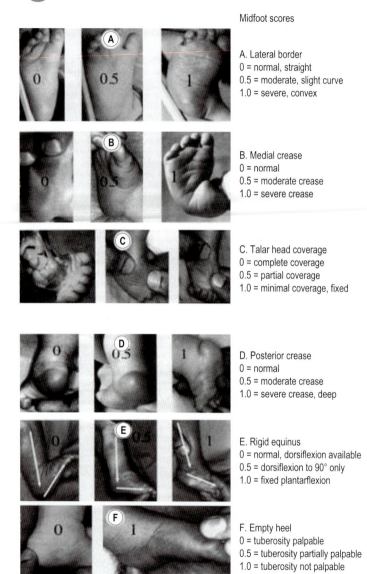

Midfoot scores

A. Lateral border
0 = normal, straight
0.5 = moderate, slight curve
1.0 = severe, convex

B. Medial crease
0 = normal
0.5 = moderate crease
1.0 = severe crease

C. Talar head coverage
0 = complete coverage
0.5 = partial coverage
1.0 = minimal coverage, fixed

D. Posterior crease
0 = normal
0.5 = moderate crease
1.0 = severe crease, deep

E. Rigid equinus
0 = normal, dorsiflexion available
0.5 = dorsiflexion to 90° only
1.0 = fixed plantarflexion

F. Empty heel
0 = tuberosity palpable
0.5 = tuberosity partially palpable
1.0 = tuberosity not palpable

Figure 8.1 Pirani scoring method. Each of the six criteria is scored 0, 0.5, 1.0. A score of 0 indicates normal findings, 0.5 shows moderate or partial deformity and 1.0 indicates severe deformity. The total Pirani score is 6, with two sub-scores for the midfoot and hindfoot scoring 3 each.

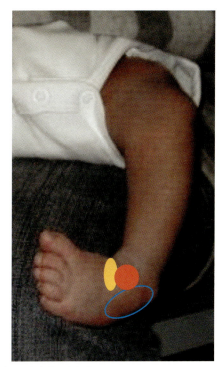

Figure 8.2 Gentle manipulation of the foot.

    d. Other scoring systems (e.g. Dimeglio) are also available (van Mulken et al 2001).

    e. The Pirani score is used at every cast change to monitor progress.

3. Manipulate to the correct position for the first cast (Fig. 8.2), repeated each 5–7 days (Morcuende et al 2005) until foot position is corrected, which usually takes approximately five to six casts (Fig. 8.3). Gentle manipulation of the foot first requires location of the head of talus (red) on the lateral side. The method of doing this

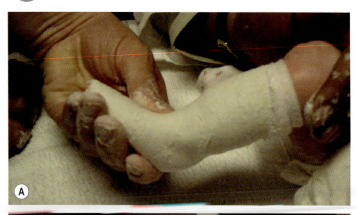

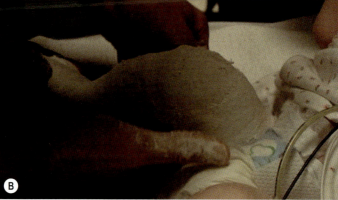

Figure 8.3 (A) Apply cast in two sections: first, foot and leg to below the knee (note the maintained manipulated foot position until the plaster has set firm). Check the first section of the cast before applying the second to ensure it achieves adequate correction of the foot. (B) Apply cast in two sections: second, connecting knee and thigh with above-knee cast, which extends to the groin. The knee is flexed at 90° and needs to be reinforced to avoid breakage.

is to: palpate the tibial and fibular malleoli with one hand, holding toes and metatarsals with the other hand. Slide thumb and forefinger from malleoli to the front of the ankle mortise. The navicular (orange) is small (forming) and, being medially displaced, will be found under the medial malleolus. The anterior calcaneus (blue) will be felt just below the talar head. Stabilize the head of the talus laterally so the foot can be abducted around the talus. Do not touch the calcaneus for this movement.

a. The arch cavus is corrected at the same time as reducing the forefoot adduction. This is achieved by inverting (supinating) and abducting the forefoot to align with the hindfoot (Morcuende et al 1994). The ankle equinus is corrected last (usually with a tenotomy).

b. To avoid upsetting or cutting the infant, cast saws are not used. Instead, it is recommended that all casts are soaked off 1 hour before the next cast is to be applied.

4. Most cases require an Achilles tenotomy to gain full correction of the ankle equinus (Fig. 8.4).

a. The ends of the severed tendon have been found to appose again within 3 weeks (Barker & Lavy 2006).

b. Analytical radiography following the tenotomy procedure in clubfeet has demonstrated a reduction of the angle between the tibia and the calcaneus (i.e. the calcaneus is less retracted) and unchanged relationship between the tibia and the talus (i.e. prevented iatrogenic rocker-bottom foot) (de Gheldere & Docquier 2008).

5. A final abductory cast is then applied for a further 3 weeks.

a. Maintain the correction using an abduction brace for 3–5 years to prevent relapse of the deformity (Fig. 8.5).

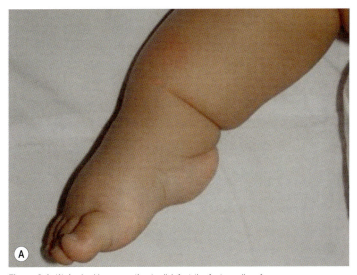

Figure 8.4 (A) Apply skin preparation to disinfect the foot on all surfaces.

Continued

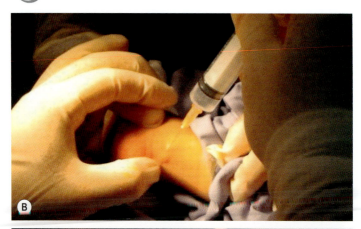

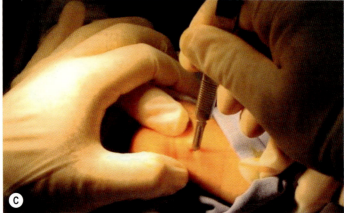

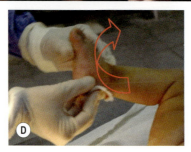

Figure 8.4 *Continued.* (B) Use a small amount (0.5 ml) of local anaesthetic solution or topical anaesthetic.
(C) Using a no. 11 or no. 15 blade, a small incision is made 1.0–1.5 cm above the calcaneus, while the foot is held in dorsiflexion.
(D) As the tendon releases, a 'pop' is felt/heard and 10–20° dorsiflexion should be gained. The 'gap' between the severed tendon ends can be palpated. A final cast is applied after the Achilles tenotomy and remains for 3 weeks. The cast must be applied with the foot abducted 60–70°. Following the removal of this final cast 20–30° of ankle dorsiflexion should be possible. The foot is now ready for splinting, which must begin immediately to avoid loss of any correction.

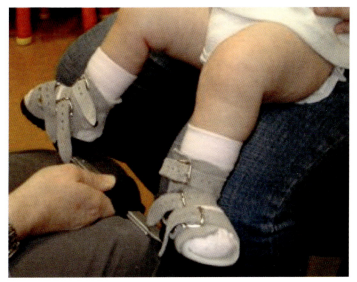

Figure 8.5 The use of the foot abduction brace is essential to prevent relapses. Many brace types are available, e.g. Steenbeck, Denis Browne and Mitchell (pictured).

  b. It has been shown that insufficient use of the brace accounts for more than 80% of relapses (Haft et al 2007; Morcuende et al 2004, 2005).
6. It is vital that children are monitored regularly.
  a. Suggested monitoring times from the initial fitting of the brace (when it is worn 23 hours/day) are: 2 weeks, 1 month, 3 months. After 3 months brace use is reduced to 16 hours/day. Continue to check every 3 months until the child is 12 months old

(depending upon the age the whole process began), 3–6 monthly checks until the child is 5–6 years old and then 6–12 monthly until age 15 years or skeletally mature.

Bearing in mind the genetically driven tendency of the clubfoot to be deformed, bracing and monitoring must be very diligent until the child is at least 5–6 years of age and beyond (Ponseti et al 2003). The parents need to be informed of the importance of the brace use right from the start of managing the clubfoot.

Relapsing clubfoot – what to watch for

- Reduced abduction.
- Reduced ankle dorsiflexion.
- Increased metatarsal adduction.
- Gait: heel varus, forefoot supination.

Relapsing clubfoot – what to do

- Re-cast, re-brace.
- For equinus: cast; may need another tenotomy, cast and splint.
- For gait supination: may need tibialis anterior transfer (to third cuneiform).

Research

Investigative findings support the Ponseti method as the best choice for initial clubfoot management. The results of research investigating the efficacy of the Ponseti method are summarized and presented in Table 8.1. The main features are that initial correction rates following casting (and tenotomy if required) are good, ranging from 70 to 100%. The other major finding is that the relapse rate is reported to directly correlate with compliance with the foot abduction brace post casting. Clearly the use of the brace is paramount if long-term results are to be achieved and parents must be educated and supported to improve compliance. These results illustrate very clearly why the Ponseti method has now grown to be the technique of choice across the world.

Key Concepts

The correct use of the Ponseti technique has been shown repeatedly to radically reduce the rate of extensive corrective surgical procedures for clubfoot (Morcuende et al 2004) and has been found to be adaptable to successful use in the developing world (Gupta et al 2006, Ponseti et al 2003, Tindall et al 2005).

Table 8.1 Research findings of the success rate of the Ponseti technique over 27 years (1980–2007)

The main features are that initial correction rates following casting (and tenotomy if required) are good, ranging from 70 to 100%. The other major finding is that the relapse rate is reported to directly correlate with compliance with the foot abduction brace post casting. Clearly the use of the brace is paramount if long-term results are to be achieved and parents must be educated and supported to improve compliance.

Author	Number of patients	Average age of patients	Number of clubfeet	Initial correction	Comment
Laaveg & Ponseti 1980	70	<6 months	104	88.5	
Ponseti et al 1981	32	Infant	32	87.5	
Cooper & Dietz 1995	45	<4 months	71	78	
Herzenberg et al 2002	27	<3 months	34	97	RCT: 3% required PMR vs 94% in control group
Lehman et al 2003	63	10.8 weeks	87	92	Correction reduced to 50% if brace not used properly
Morcuende et al 2004	157	Most <6 months	256	98	Relapses due to poor brace use
Dobbs et al 2004	51	12 weeks	86	100	Relapses (31%) correlate with brace use: 183 times increased recurrence risk
Thacker et al 2005	30	<6 months	44	70	Brace use avoids relapse
Tindall et al 2005	75	11.5 weeks	100	98	Malawi study
Morcuende et al 2005	230	3–5 months	319	92–93	Brace use improves results
Gupta et al 2006	96	Babies	154	100	India study
Changulani et al 2006	66		100	96	Relapses due to poor brace use
Shack & Eastwood 2007	24	3 weeks	40	97.5	Physical therapist delivered treatment
Ponseti et al 2006	50	3 months	75	100	Complex clubfeet, 14% relapse with poor brace use
Goksan et al 2006	92		134	97	Relapses due to poor brace use, previous treatment, doctor's experience
Haft et al 2007	51	15 days	73	100	Relapses (41%) correlate with brace use

The 'Feet for Walking' clubfoot project

The 'Feet for Walking' clubfoot project commenced in 2004 (www.feetforwalking.org).

Many seminars have been run in provinces in central Vietnam to provide education to hospital and clinic staff (Evans & Thanh, 2008). The International Red Cross (ICRC) convened seminars for doctors in Ho Chi Minh City in central Vietnam in 2007–08 for the Ponseti technique to be further conveyed to doctors and physical therapists. The first training seminar in the Ponseti method was held in Bangladesh in 2008 as a further initiative of the ICRC. It is apparent that many older children have been neglected and children aged 4–6 years with untreated clubfeet are commonly seen. This situation is documented in research from Brazil, where the Ponseti method has been successfully modified to give good results, if over a longer treatment course (Lourenco & Morcuende 2007). Many similar projects are operating in other developing nations.

References

Barker SL, Lavy CBD 2006 Correlation of clinical and ultrasonographic findings after Achilles tenotomy in idiopathic club foot. Journal of Bone and Joint Surgery – British Volume 88(3):377–379

Changulani M, Garg NK, Rajagopal TS et al 2006 Treatment of idiopathic clubfoot using the Ponseti method: initial experience. Journal of Bone and Joint Surgery – British Volume 88(10):1385–1387

Cooper DM, Dietz FR 1995 Treatment of idiopathic clubfoot. Journal of Bone and Joint Surgery – American Volume 77(10):1477–1489

de Gheldere A, Docquier P-L 2008 Analytical radiography of clubfoot after tenotomy. Journal of Pediatric Orthopaedics 28(6):691–694

Dobbs MB, Rudzki JR, Purcell DB et al 2004 Factors predictive of outcome after use of the Ponseti method for the treatment of idiopathic clubfeet. Journal of Bone and Joint Surgery – American Volume 86(1):22–27

Dobbs MB, Nunley R, Schoenecker PL 2006 Long-term follow-up of patients with clubfeet treated with extensive soft-tissue release. Journal of Bone and Joint Surgery – American Volume 88(5):986–996

Dyer PJ, De Vaus DA 2006 The role of the Pirani scoring system in the management of club foot by the Ponseti method. Journal of Bone and Joint Surgery – British Volume 88(8):1082–1084

Evans AM 2007 Pirani severity scoring for the clubfoot program in Vietnam: a reliability study. 22nd Australasian Podiatry Conference Book of Abstracts [May], 73 [Abstract]

Evans AM, Do Van Thanh 2008 The management of infant clubfoot deformity in Vietnam, using Ponseti method. Revue Médicale 2008: 1–19

Evans AM, Do Van Thanh 2009 A review of the Ponseti method and development of an infant clubfoot program in Vietnam. Journal of the American Podiatric Medical Association 99(4):306–316

Goksan SB, Bursali A, Biligi F et al 2006 Ponseti technique for the correction of idiopathic clubfeet presenting up to 1 year of age: a preliminary study in children with untreated or complex deformities. Archives of Orthopaedic and Trauma Surgery 126(1):15–21

Gupta A, Singh S, Patel P et al 2006 Evaluation of the utility of the Ponseti method of correction of clubfoot deformity in a developing nation. International Orthopedics 32(1):75–79

Haft GF, Walker CG, Craxford AD 2007 Early clubfoot recurrence after use of the Ponseti method in a New Zealand population. Journal of Bone and Joint Surgery – American Volume 89(3):487–493

Herzenberg JE, Radler C, Bor N 2002 Ponseti versus traditional methods of casting for idiopathic clubfoot. Journal of Pediatric Orthopedics 22(4):517–521

Laaveg SJ, Ponseti IV 1980 Long term results of treatment of congenital club foot. Journal of Bone and Joint Surgery – American Volume 62(1):23–31

Lehman WB, Mohaideen A, Madan S et al 2003 A method for the early evaluation of the Ponseti (Iowa) technique for the treatment of idiopathic clubfoot. Journal of Pediatric Orthopedics B 12(2): 133–140

Lourenco AF, Morcuende JA 2007 Correction of neglected idiopathic club foot by the Ponseti method. Journal of Bone and Joint Surgery – British Volume 89B(3):378–381

Agarwal RA, Pandey S 2007 Step by step management of clubfoot by Ponseti technique. Jaypee Brothers, New Delhi, India

Morcuende JA, Weinstein SL, Dietz FR et al 1994 Plaster cast treatment of clubfoot: the Ponseti method of manipulation and casting. Journal of Pediatric Orthopedics B 3(2):161–167

Morcuende JA, Dolan LA, Dietz FR et al 2004 Radical reduction in the rate of extensive corrective surgery for clubfoot using the Ponseti method. Pediatrics 113(2):376–380

Morcuende JA, Abbasi D, Dolan LA et al 2005 Results of an accelerated Ponseti protocol for clubfoot. Journal of Pediatric Orthopedics 25(5):623–626

Pandey S, Pandey AK 2003 The classification of clubfoot: a practical approach. The Foot 13:61–65

Pirani S, Zeznick L, Hodges D 2001 Magnetic resonance imaging study of the congenital clubfoot treated with the Ponseti method. Journal of Pediatric Orthopedics 21(6):719–726

Ponseti IV 1997 Common errors in the treatment of congenital clubfoot. International Orthopedics 21:137–141

Ponseti IV, El-Khoury GY, Ippolito E et al 1981 A radiographic study of skeletal deformities in treated clubfeet. Clinical Orthopaedics and Related Research 160:30–42

Ponseti IV, Morcuende JA, Mosca V et al 2003 Clubfoot: Ponseti management, 2nd edn. Global HELP Publication. Online. Available at: http://www.global-help.org/publications/books/book_cfponseti.html (accessed 4 May 2009)

Ponseti IV, Zhivkov M, Davis N et al 2006 Treatment of the complex idiopathic clubfoot. Clinical Orthopaedics and Related Research 451: 171–176

Shack N, Eastwood DM 2007 Early results of a physiotherapist-delivered Ponseti service for the management of idiopathic congenital talipes equinovarus foot deformity. Journal of Bone and Joint Surgery – British Volume 88(8):1085–1089

Tachdjian MO 1985 The child's foot. WB Saunders, Philadelphia

Thacker MM, Scher DM, Sala DM et al 2005 Use of the foot abduction orthosis following Ponseti casts: is it essential? Journal of Pediatric Orthopedics 25(2):225–228

Tindall Aj, Steinlechner CWB, Lavy CBD 2005 Results of manipulation of idiopathic clubfoot deformity in Malawi by orthopaedic clinical officers using the Ponseti method. Journal of Pediatric Orthopedics 25(5):627–629

van Mulken JMJ, Bulstra SK, Hoefnagels HM 2001 Evaluation of the treatment of clubfeet with the Dimeglio score. Journal of Pediatrics 21(5):642–647

Further reading

Ponseti IV, Morcuende JA, Mosca V et al 2009 Clubfoot: Ponseti management, 3rd edn.

The reader is strongly encouraged to access this publication, which can be downloaded free from: www.global-help.org

Ponseti International Association website: http://www.ponseti.info/v1/

Steps charity, which assists children born with orthopaedic problems, website: http://www.steps-charity.org.uk/

Metatarsus adductus

Introduction

Historically metatarsus adductus (MTA) was first described in Germany in the mid 19th century and only acknowledged in the English literature for the first time in 1921 (Berg 1986, Kite 1967). At times synonymous with *metatarsus varus*, MTA has long been a controversial entity in terms of treatment. In part, this confusion has been due to inconsistent identification of sub-types and thus a lack of helpful classification. Different types of MTA need to be identified as these need to be managed, and respond differently to treatment (Dietz 1994, Ganley 1984, Gore & Spencer 2004, Ponseti & Becker 1966, Sass & Hassan 2003). Fortunately the difficult types of MTA are in the minority and the clinical course is generally one of natural improvement (Widhe 1997). However, the less numerous, recalcitrant sub-types of MTA need to be carefully screened and managed to avert ongoing problems as the child grows (Gore & Spencer 2004; Sass & Hassan 2003; Tachdjian 1985, 1997).

Aetiology

Metatarsus adductus is defined as a transverse plane deformity at Lisfranc's (the tarso-metatarso) joint in which the metatarsals and phalanges adduct from the rear foot, giving rise to a convex lateral border (Gore & Spencer 2004; Shepherd 1995; Tachdjian 1985, 1997; Tax 1980; Thomson 1993; Valmassy 1996).

The most cited causative factor is abnormal intrauterine position and resulting compression from the uterine wall against the developing foot (Valmassy 1996). Limited histological research from the second trimester has indicated abnormality of the medial cuneiform (Morcuende & Ponseti 1996). Other associations include (alone or in combination):

- tight abductor hallucis
- malpositioned tibialis anterior tendon at the base of the first ray
- tibialis anterior contracture (with weak peroneals)
- abnormal insertion of tibialis posterior
- arrested foot development in the first trimester (Valmassy 1996).

Prevalence

Metatarsus adductus is estimated to occur in 1:1000 births, making it a common foot deformity (Dietz 1994, Gore & Spencer 2004, Sass & Hassan 2003).

Twenty years ago, Berg reported that 56% of children referred to a particular institution in the USA had a diagnosis of metatarsus adductus (Berg 1986).

MTA has been reportedly more frequent in females, showing a predisposition for the left foot (Sass & Hassan 2003), yet others state there is no gender predilection (Valmassy 1996).

Some 50% of cases are bilateral and there is a 5% chance of subsequent siblings of affected children also having MTA (Drennan 1992).

Diagnosis

The diagnosis of MTA is clinical and includes a tell-tale 'C'-shaped or 'banana' foot appearance. The small feet of neonates presenting with MTA morphology need to be carefully examined and classified, so that treatment is not withheld from the (fewer) types which do not otherwise resolve.

Key *Concepts*

MTA can be usefully classified by three main attributes:

1. type
2. flexibility
3. degree of deformity (Ganley 1984, 1991).

Classification

Classification by type

Metatarsus adductus is a broad generic term, used to describe a range of congenital foot deformities (Morcuende & Ponseti 1996). Clinically it is useful to sub-type MTA as follows:

1. Developmental metatarsus adductus (MTA type 1)

The developmental or postural type of MTA is positional in nature due to tightness of abductor hallucis, which may have been congenitally tight or as a result of intrauterine moulding. Fortunately this is the most common type of MTA and can usually be expected to spontaneously resolve. Manual stretching of the foot to a corrected posture at nappy changes may hasten this resolve. The metatarsals are in normal alignment and the adduction of the hallux (*atavism*) is only seen in dynamic simulated weight-bearing situations. The lateral border is typically straight.

2. True metatarsus adductus (MTA type 2)

This is the simplest of the structural types exhibiting transverse plane adduction of the forefoot on rear foot. All metatarsals are adducted, with the first being most adducted and the fifth being least adducted. The adduction is isolated at the Lisfranc joint (tarso-metatarso) and results in the 'banana' or 'C'-shaped foot. The midfoot and rear foot are relatively normal (Drennan 1992).

3. Metatarsus (adducto) varus (MTA type 3)

This foot shows transverse plane adduction and also frontal plane inversion of the forefoot on rear foot. It involves all metatarsals being adducted at the Lisfranc joint and inverted distally. The calcaneus is generally everted, but can be straight. This type of MTA usually becomes a more entrenched deformity with time, so must be both recognized and treated effectively (Bleck 1971, Valmassy 1996).

4. Skew foot (MTA type 4)

This more complicated and – prognosis-wise – worse foot has transverse plane adduction and also frontal plane inversion of the forefoot on rear foot. Simultaneously, the rear foot is everted at both subtalar and midtarsal joints. This is a complex foot type, which in an older child or adult exhibits lateral midtarsal shift on X-ray. This type of MTA is usually acquired as either a compensation for uncorrected metatarsus varus (type 3) or severe true metatarsus adductus (type 2), but may also be induced by

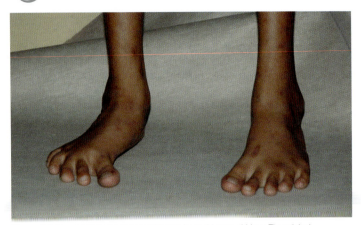

Figure 9.1 Uncorrected metatarsus adductus in an 11-year-old boy. The original transverse plane deformity found in types 2 and 3 has progressed to the serpentine or skew foot (type 4).

inappropriate treatment, for example forcibly abducting the forefoot without stabilizing the rear foot (Fig. 9.1; Ganley 1984).

Most importantly, you must notice that none of these deformities has a sagittal plane component, which if present will identify it as talipes equinovarus or 'clubfoot'. Metatarsus adductus has been loosely termed 'a third of a club-foot' but does not exhibit ankle equinus (Ganley 1984, Kite 1967).

Classification by flexibility and degree of deformity

1. Flexibility

This is assessed by reducing the adduction of the forefoot on a stable rear foot in the transverse plane:

- Flexible: the deformity will reduce with ease, it being possible to abduct the forefoot beyond the foot's midline.
- Reduced flexibility: the deformity will reduce no further than the foot's midline with passive abductory force.
- Rigid: the deformity will not reduce and with abductory force applied, remains adducted, i.e. it does not reach the foot's midline.

To determine overall flexibility it is also necessary to check the tension of abductor hallucis in both non-weight-bearing and also weight-bearing (simulated if baby is pre-walking). It is common with a tight abductor hallucis belly to see a flexible metatarsus adductus exhibit marked adduction of the hallux in weight-bearing and gait. This may be termed *dynamic hallux varus* or an *atavistic first ray.*

Clinical flexibility guides treatment. Structurally fixed cases will not reduce passively and may require surgical correction.

2. Degree of deformity

Bleck's (1983) simple clinical scale records the severity of metatarsus adductus from the child's footprint. The heel is bisected and a line extended through the forefoot (Fig. 9.2). Bleck's scale can be adapted for clinical use as shown below. Clinically, the use of a ruler is useful for this method.

This method allows for simple non-invasive baseline assessment and monitoring of the MTA deformity and classification of the degree of deformity:

i.	normal	heel bisection ends distally at	2nd/3rd toes
ii.	mild	heel bisection ends distally at	3rd toe
iii.	moderate	heel bisection ends distally at	3rd/4th toes
iv.	severe	heel bisection ends distally at	4th/5th toes laterally.

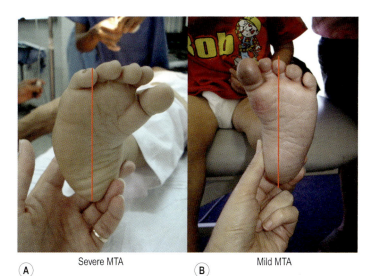

A	Severe MTA	**B**	Mild MTA

Figure 9.2 (A) Severe metatarsus adductus.
(B) Mild metatarsus adductus.

Differential diagnosis

- Clubfoot (talipes equinovarus).
- Metatarsus primus varus.
- Cerebral palsy.

Typical clinical picture

Examination

Examination and diagnosis of metatarsus adductus is based on clinical appearance in the infant and young child. The prominence of the styloid process of the fifth metatarsal is a hallmark sign for adduction of all five metatarsals versus the so-called atavistic first ray where the lateral border of the foot is straight but the medial concave/adducted. Skin creasing on the medial side is usually associated with a less flexible MTA deformity which is more likely to require treatment. There should be no reduction of ankle joint dorsiflexion with MTA. If ankle range is reduced, you need to suspect talipes equinovarus or clubfoot.

Key Concepts

Atavistic first ray refers to a primitive foot type where the first ray acts more like a thumb with grasping ability. Useful for hanging from trees originally, this can clinically contribute to an increased or 'dynamic' MTA with weight-bearing where the first ray adducts and can medially rotate the lower leg and contribute to an intoeing gait. Shoes with a straight medial border seem to reduce the action of abductor hallucis and in turn reduce the hallux adduction grasp and intoeing.

Radiological examination is useful in later stages to classify the extent of deformity based on specific joint angle deviations and values (Table 9.1).

1. Clinical findings

In the very young child (less than 6 months) it is most useful to look at the foot from the plantar aspect, placing the small foot between the index finger and thumb such that the index finger aligns with the lateral border of the foot to act as a 'ruler' (Fig. 9.3).

In this position:

- observe the position of the hallux compared to the medial border
- observe the shape of the lateral border
- look at rear foot alignment
- assess frontal plane position of forefoot to rear foot.

Table 9.1 X-ray angles pertinent to metatarsus adductus deformity in the older child

Angle		Normal values
Metatarsus adductus angle (AP)	Angle formed between longitudinal bisection of second metatarsal and the midtarsal divide The midfoot divide is difficult to identify prior to ossification	Birth: 22–25° Toddler:15–20° Adult: 10°
Talo-first metatarsal angle (AP)	Angle formed between talar bisection and first metatarsal bisection Useful as a basic evaluation of atavistic first metatarsal versus forefoot adductus	0–20°
Talo-calcaneal angle (AP)	Angle formed between talar and calcaneal bisections Useful in discrimination from clubfoot Usually is normal in metatarsus adductus but may be higher angle in skew foot and lower angle in clubfoot	20–40°
Calaneo-cuboid angle (lateral)	Angle formed between lateral aspect of cuboid and the calcaneus pitch This angle may be increased in skew foot type	0–5°

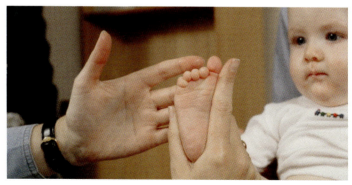

Figure 9.3 Clinical assessment of metatarsus adductus. The cleft between the examiner's thumb and forefinger is utilized to assess the adduction of both the medial and lateral foot borders.

Key Concepts

Classify the foot with respect to:

- Type: 1, 2, 3 or 4.
- Flexibility: flexible, reduced, rigid.
- Degree of deformity: normal, mild, moderate, severe (Bleck scale).

It may be useful to photograph the foot or take a paper tracing for future reference. This is non-invasive, safe and retrospectively valuable. Bleck's scale can be applied to a weight-bearing tracing (for older infants) to assess the degree of deformity. This can be very helpful in discussions with parents and other practitioners (see Fig. 9.2).

2. Radiological findings

Diagnosis of this entity is primarily clinical as described above. It is not necessary or helpful to use radiology to diagnose metatarsus adductus in infancy, as the foot is largely chondral in architecture. It may be of use if treatment is not effective or to check for secondary compensations in toddlers and older children.

X-ray examination is useful in the severe, rigid or skew foot varieties of metatarsus adductus. It can, in these cases, help to differentiate metatarsus adductus from talipes equinovarus (clubfoot).

Standard radiological techniques (as employed for adults) are inappropriate as the midtarsal region is cartilaginous in the young child or infant. Views need to be taken by taping the foot/feet to the film plate to give simulated weight-bearing. AP and lateral views are utilized.

Angles and range values are as described in Table 9.1.

Associations

Metatarsus adductus has been both associated and disassociated with congenital dislocations of developmental dysplasia of the hip (Drennan 1992, Wenger & Leach 1986). It is generally accepted that careful examination of the hips of babies be performed, rather than routine pelvic X-rays (Drennan 1992).

There is also cited association between metatarsus adductus, reduced tibial torsion (medial) and intoeing gait (Cusick 1990, Dietz 1994, Killam 1989, Li & Leong 1999, Wells 1996). A radiographic study of 100 feet showed MTA in 55% of cases with hallux valgus compared to 19% of subjects without hallux valgus (Ferrari & Malone-Lee 2003). In a case controlled study, juvenile hallux valgus has been associated with an increased metatarsus primus adductus angle but not definitively associated with MTA (McCluney & Tinley 2006).

Treatment

There is much controversy regarding the treatment or non-treatment of metatarsus adductus. According to one author results are better when treated before 8 months of age (Sass & Hassan 2003). Others cite 6% spontaneous resolution in 130 feet (Widhe 1997). Only 11% of 379 children required treatment (Dietz 1994). Advocates of non-treatment often acknowledge some residual deformity but feel the rate is low and thus this is acceptable. Cited residue includes:

- cosmesis
- shoe fit
- early hallux valgus
- ball and socket ankle (Tachdjian 1985).

In most studies supportive of non-treatment only clinical appearance was used to assess correction. This may mean that:

- Children with excessive subtalar and/or midtarsal joint pronation may 'disguise' their remaining deformity (but create a *skew foot,* i.e. rear foot everted, forefoot adducted, metatarsophalangeal joints abducted).
- Shoe use will abduct toes to give appearance of correction.
- Partial correction has occurred.

However, a recent study found the incidence of foot deformity to be 4% in 2401 newborns, of which 75% were various forms of adductus types. This study found that by age 6 years 87% had resolved and by 16 years 95% had resolved (Widhe 1997). This is a powerful argument for non-treatment in the main, but the real issues are: (i) to detect those feet with metatarsus adductus which will not resolve, and (ii) to ensure that metatarsus adductus initially assessed to be resolving is monitored (reducing later problematic instances). The general consensus in paediatric orthopaedic texts is that treatment is required when 'significant' deformity exists or persists after 3–4 months of age, i.e. when spontaneous correction following release from uterine confinement has not occurred by this time (Valmassy 1996). This has been supported by a randomized controlled trial of 41 feet with metatarsus adductus (in 25 babies) which addressed moderate and severe types (Bleck scale criteria). This study, which provides best current evidence, found that two types of abducting foot orthoses (static, dynamic) improved the metatarsus adductus deformity. This trial also recommended treatment of the moderate and severe metatarsus adductus foot types before 8 months of age for best results (Camin et al 2004).

Table 9.2 When and how I treat MTA in infants

MTA type	Flexibility* – flexible – moderate – reduced	Bleck scale** – moderate – severe	Age 4–8 months	Age >10 months	Age walking +
1	Postural MTA resolves – no treatment required				
2	Serial casts/abduction orthoses to correct Splint/shoes to maintain correction (if flexible, moderate may use Wheaton brace or other splint as primary method)		Cast, especially if reduced flexibility/ severe. Straight/ reverse last shoes by day and night splint	Consider 1–2 initial casts; straight/ reverse last shoes/ in-shoe wedge or orthoses and night splint
3	Serial casts/abduction orthoses to correct Splint/shoes to maintain correction				
4	Skew foot: can manage with specific shoe selection, foot orthoses, surgery				

*Flexibility: rigid MTA requires a surgical opinion.
**Bleck scale: I usually leave 'mild' MTA or use straight last shoes once walking.

The author's approach to metatarsus adductus management is summarized in Table 9.2.

Treatment options basically divide into conservative versus surgical options. Only a brief overview will be provided here. Further detail is readily available in both texts and journals.

Conservative

- Passive stretching and massage: for *mild* flexible cases (type 1).

The following methods are indicated for MTA types 2 and 3, which rate as *moderate* or *severe* on the Bleck footprint scale.

- Serial plaster of Paris casting: incorporating prior stretching. This is the standard treatment approach where the foot is cast in a progressively corrected posture with casts being changed every 1–2 weeks for 6–8 weeks. It is usually necessary to follow this treatment with a night splint for at least 6–8 weeks to maintain the cast correction (Fig. 9.4).

- Abduction foot orthoses: supported by a clinical trial these orthoses best correct moderate and severe MTA when treatment is commenced before 8 months of age. The clinical trial also advocated the

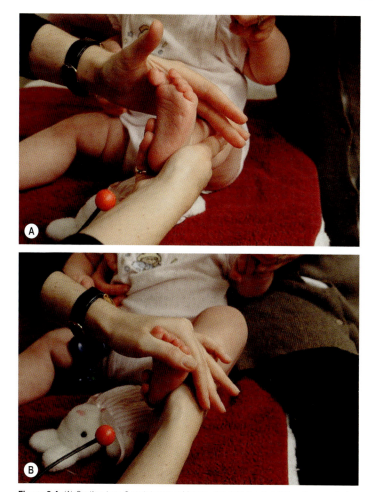

Figure 9.4 (A) Casting type 3 metatarsus adductus: the right hand stabilizes the rear foot over the TNJ (talo-navicular joint) medially and CCJ (calcaneo-cuboid joint) laterally. (B) The left hand abducts the forefoot, everting the forefoot as necessary.

Continued

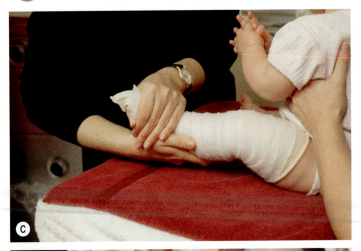

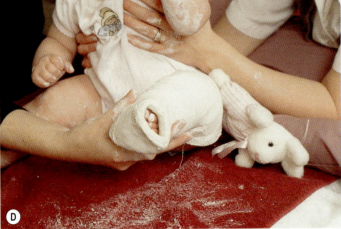

Figure 9.4 *Continued*. (C) After this manipulation is held for a minute, padding and then plaster are applied.
(D) The same corrective hand holds are used until the cast is set.

further use of reverse last shoes in cases where correction was incomplete (Camin et al 2004).

- Splinting: can be used as a first-line approach in milder cases (instead of serial casting) or as a subsequent corrective device following the use of serial casting in more severe cases. There are many splints available, all with particular advantages and disadvantages. Summarized in Chapter 15, these include:
  - Ganley splint
  - Denis Browne bar
  - Unibar
  - Counter-rotation system
  - Fillauer bar.
  - Wheaton brace (only one not requiring shoes; Fig. 9.5). This pre-formed brace can be very useful for the management of

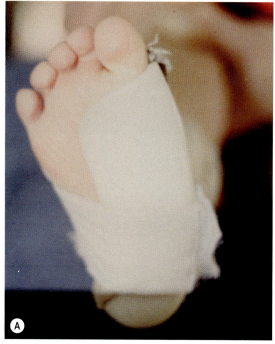

Figure 9.5 (A) The Wheaton brace.

Continued

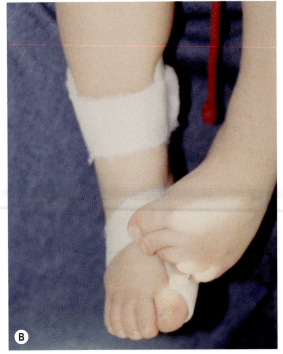

Figure 9.5 *Continued.* (B) The Wheaton brace.

MTA. Unlike all other splints and braces, no shoes are required. The sizing is sometimes too specific for chubby legs and little feet, but can be carefully heat adjusted. Alternatively a similar effect can be achieved using aquaplast, as for an ankle-foot orthosis or an abducting foot.

Surgical

- For cases not amenable to conservative options or following failed conservative management.
- Soft tissue procedures:
  - utilize in younger children before midfoot ossification has occurred
  - may include: abductor hallucis tenotomy; tarso-metatarso ligamentous release (2–7-year-olds).

- Osseous procedures:
  - chondrotomy of lesser metatarsal bases with casting (6–8-year-olds)
  - osteotomies of lesser metatarsal bases and also osteotomy of first metatarsal distal to the physis. This will include internal fixation to hold the correction (over 8 years of age)
  - open wedge reduction osteotomy of first cuneiform (6–8-year-olds)
  - cuboid wedge reduction osteotomy with internal fixation.

Evidence-based management

Defining the type of MTA helps the clinician to decide whether or not to treat MTA. Remember that type 1 (the most common type) appears to resolve in time, while types 2 and 4 (moderate to severe on Bleck's foot-print scale) have been shown to correct with the use of abduction foot orthoses (best used before 8 months of age; Table 9.3).

Remember the basic steps to managing children with metatarsus adductus. These are:

1. Be sure of the diagnosis – do not miss a clubfoot.
2. Use the best evidence available for management – abductory foot orthoses for moderate to severe (types 2 and 3) MTA, ideally treating before 8 months of age.
3. Monitor treatment outcomes – Bleck's footprint scale, X-rays.
4. Re-visit differential diagnoses and seek medical investigations if clinical picture changes from definition (Fig. 9.6).

Table 9.3

	Evidence hierarchy	Interventions
	Systematic review	None
	Randomized controlled trial	Abduction foot orthoses
	Cohort	None
	Case control	None
	Case series	Serial casting, surgery
	Non-rating studies	Serial casting, splints, boots, surgery

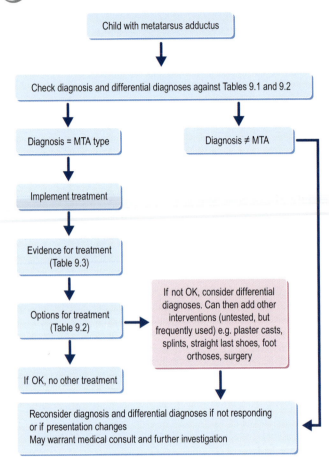

Figure 9.6 Algorithm to guide metatarsus adductus management.

References

Berg EE 1986 A reappraisal of metatarsus adductus and skewfoot. Journal of Bone and Joint Surgery – American Volume 68(8):1185–1196

Bleck EE 1971 The shoeing of children: sham or science? Developmental Medicine and Child Neurology 13(2):188–195

Bleck EE 1983 Metatarsus adductus: classification and relationship to outcome of treatment. Journal of Pediatric Orthopedics 3:2

Camin M, Vangelista A, Cosentino A et al 2004 Early and delayed orthotic treatment in congenital metatarsus varus: effectiveness of two types of orthoses. Europa Medicophysica 40(4):285–291

Cusick BD 1990 Progressive casting and splinting for lower extremity deformities in children with neuromotor dysfunction. Therapy Skill Builders, Arizona

Dietz FR 1994 Intoeing – fact, fiction and opinion. American Family Physician 50(6):1249–1264

Drennan JC 1992 The child's foot and ankle. Raven Press, New York

Ferrari J, Malone-Lee J 2003 A radiographic study of the relationship between metatarsus adductus and hallux valgus. Journal of Foot and Ankle Surgery 42(1):9–14

Ganley JV 1984 Corrective casting in infants. Clinics in Podiatry 1(3):501–516

Ganley JV 1991 The hopscotch position: a screening test. Journal of the American Podiatric Medical Association 81(3):136

Gore AI, Spencer JP 2004 The newborn foot. American Family Physician 69(4):865–872

Killam PE 1989 Orthopaedic assessment of young children: developmental variations. Nurse Practitioner 14(7):27–36

Kite JH 1967 Errors and complications in treating foot conditions in children. Clinical Orthopaedics and Related Research 53:31–38

Li YH, Leong JCY 1999 Intoeing gait in children. Hong Kong Medical Journal 5(4):360–366

McCluney JG, Tinley P 2006 Radiographic measurements of patients with juvenile hallux valgus compared with age-matched controls: a cohort investigation. Journal of Foot and Ankle Surgery 45(3):161–167

Morcuende JA, Ponseti IV 1996 Congenital metatarsus adductus in early human fetal development. Clinical Orthopaedics and Related Research (333):261–266

Ponseti IV, Becker JR 1966 Congenital metatarsus adductus: the results of treatment. Journal of Bone and Joint Surgery – American Volume 48(4):702–711

Sass P, Hassan G 2003 Lower extremity abnormalities in children. American Family Physician 68(3):461–468

Shepherd RB 1995 Physiotherapy in paediatrics, 3rd edn. Butterworth Heinemann, Oxford

Tachdjian MO 1985 The child's foot. WB Saunders, Philadelphia

Tachdjian MO 1997 Clinical pediatric orthopedics. Appleton & Lange, Stamford, CT

Tax HR 1980 Podopediatrics. Williams and Wilkins, Baltimore, p. 52

Thomson P 1993 Introduction to podopaediatrics. WB Saunders, London

Valmassy RL 1996 Clinical biomechanics of the lower extremities. Mosby, St Louis, p. 246

Wells L 1996 Common lower extremity problems in children. Orthopedics 23(2):299–303

Wenger DR, Leach J 1986 Foot deformities in infants and children. Pediatric Clinics of North America 33(6):1411–1427

Widhe T 1997 Foot deformities at birth: a londitudinal prospective study over a 16 year period. Journal of Pediatric Orthopedics 17:20–24

Further reading

Camin M, Vangelista A, Corontino A 2004 Early and delayed orthotic treatment in congenital metatarsus varus: effectiveness of two types of orthoses. Europa Medicophysica 40(4):285–291

Intoeing gait

Introduction

An intoeing walking or running gait is a frequent childhood concern that podiatrists may be asked to verify. It is important for any clinician to recognize when observable intoeing may be expected as a part of normal development and when it is clearly abnormal, causing problems and warranting intervention.

It is equally important that the child be fully assessed, beginning as always with good elicitation and recording of the clinical history. Gait and objective evaluation should be performed, always keeping the subjective history in mind. Intoeing gait is a frequent problem in cerebral palsy, which can present quite subtly in young children and always needs to be considered as a part of the differential diagnosis.

Aetiology

Intoeing gait may originate from a single cause or multiple factors (to be discussed later in this chapter) which seem to be age related (Li & Leong 1999). Most reviews agree that primary causes of intoeing gait at different ages generally follow a developmental pattern (Fabry et al 1994, Li & Leong 1999, Lincoln & Suen 2003, Sass & Hassan 2003, Weseley et al 1981, Widhe 1997):

- Infant (aged 1–2 years) – metatarsus adductus
- Toddler (aged 2–3 years) – internal tibial torsion
- Children (aged over 3 years) – femoral torsion.

Prevalence

It has been cited that 1 in 10 children aged between 2 and 5 years has an intoeing gait (Ryan 2001). Elsewhere, some 30% of children have been observed at age 4 years, with only 4% intoeing as adults (Thackeray & Beeson 1996a).

Diagnosis

While it is agreed that intoeing gait is a commonly reported problem in children, there remains much opinion and less science about its significance as a clinical finding (Fixsen & Valman 1981, Lincoln & Suen 2003, Valmassy 1996).

Key *Concepts*

The basic diagnosis of intoeing is easy as the child is seen to walk with an adducted angle of gait. The significance of an adducted foot progression angle has been contentious, but numerous investigations agree that intoeing generally reduces with age (see Table 10.1; Fabry et al 1994, Lincoln & Suen 2003, Ryan 2001, Thackeray & Beeson 1996a, Wenger & Leach 1986, Weseley et al 1981, Widhe 1997).

Differential diagnosis

If intoeing gait is not developmental, consider familial, neurological and orthopaedic factors.

Developmental factors

As can be seen from Table 10.1, most forms of intoeing gait are developmental and resolve with increasing age. Intoeing gait in children which is functionally disabling, painful, increasing over time, associated with a limp or presents a very asymmetrical gait pattern requires closer attention, investigation and perhaps treatment.

Familial factors

Familial intoeing gait patterns will usually be revealed as part of a full case history and inquiry. Developmental intoeing gait seems to be more common in the early childhood years in some families.

Table 10.1 Observations of gait angles across 25 years

The consensus is that intoeing is common in childhood to age 6 years and that the adducted angle of gait then reduces with increasing age. Clinicians must be alert to compensations which may occur to abduct the angle of gait in some cases, e.g. reduced knee extension, flat feet.

Date	Age	Angle of gait findings
1997	Birth – 16 years	By 6 years, 87%, and at 16 years, 95% of adductus deformities had resolved (Widhe 1997)
1996	4–16 years	Mean +4.2° Range −8° to +16° (Losel et al 1996)
1996	3, 6 and 9 years	25% at 3 years 33% at 6 years 7% at 9 years 8% adults (Thackeray & Beeson 1996b)
1990	4 years – adult	16% had intoeing gait 30% of 4 year olds intoe vs 4% of adults (Svenningsen et al 1990)
1974	Children	4.5% intoeing 80% correct by 8 years (Thackeray & Beeson 1996b)
1971	Children	13.6% intoeing gait (Ho et al 2000)

Neurological factors

Intoeing gait is common in children with cerebral palsy where prevalence has been reported as greater than 60% (70% in quadriplegic, 66% in diplegic, 54% in hemiplegic children) (Rethlefsen et al 2006). Medial hip rotation and medial tibial torsion are the most common causes in this population, along with a varus/cavus foot type. Spasticity of the adductors and medial hamstrings influence both gait angle and torsion of the young femurs and tibiae (Tervo et al 2002).

Key *Concepts*

In addition to an intoeing gait, cerebral palsy markers may include:

- abnormal muscle tone
- limited hip abduction
- leg length discrepancy (Li & Leong 1999)
- significant birth history (e.g. birth weight, gestational age, Apgar scores, complications) (Lincoln & Suen 2003)
- delayed walking (e.g. 16–18 months).

Any of these findings, which raise suspicion of an underlying neurological problem, should be more intensively assessed with referral to a paediatrician or paediatric orthopaedic or neurological specialist being arranged.

Orthopaedic factors

Hip dysplasia should be suspected if hip range of motion is altered or asymmetrical, or if a limp or limb length difference is evident in addition to an intoeing gait pattern.

Achondroplasia has been found to be associated with lower limb abnormalities, including reduced (lateral) tibial torsion and increased femoral (medial) torsion (Song et al 2006).

Clubfoot (talipes equinovarus) or metatarsus adductus can result in a 'C'-shaped foot and contribute to an intoeing gait pattern. It is clearly important to correctly diagnose the foot type, as both prognosis and management issues are very different (see Chs 8 and 9; Morcuende & Ponseti 1996, Morcuende et al 2004).

Typical clinical picture

Classically the child presents with an intoeing gait pattern and worried parents. While most cases of intoeing gait will be developmental, it is important to take a full and thorough history and to examine the musculoskeletal system so that any underlying disorders are detected (or at least suspected and referred for further medical evaluation) before presuming to focus on the benign rotational problem and reassure the parents (Fabry et al 1994, Li & Leong 1999, Lincoln & Suen 2003, Ryan 2001).

History

Some simple, but revealing questions may include:

- When did the parent first notice the intoe?
- Were they aware of any inward rotation of the legs or feet at birth?
- How big was the baby at birth?
- Were the hips examined and were they stable?

Check the child's milestones to get an indication of development:

- At what age did the child sit, crawl, stand and walk? Significantly delayed walking may suggest a neuromuscular disorder, e.g. cerebral palsy, hypotonia (Cusick 1990).
- Is the intoe getting better or worse over time or has it stayed the same?

- Has there been any treatment and did this change the angle of the intoe pattern?
- What positions does the child sit in, sleep in? Both sitting and sleeping postures have been thought to be of great importance to both the aetiology and management of children with intoeing gait. Perhaps a better interpretation is that these postures may act to prevent resolution of the problem as opposed to being singular causes (Redmond 2000). While it has been shown that chronic sleeping postures can deform limbs in neonates and affect later gait (Katz et al 1991), caution is advised in deeming postures as causative of intoeing gaits.
- Is there a family history of this condition?
- How are older members now with respect to pain and function?
- How much of a problem is it?
- Is it of mild aesthetic concern or is it severe and limiting the child's ability to walk and run?

Spend adequate time taking the history as this will usually guide both your examination and the management plans.

Examination

There are probably many ways of dealing with assessment of this condition. My own approach to the child presenting with an intoed gait is to run through an organized physical examination, which is focused by prior history details and gait observation.

Starting proximally (simply my preference – it does not matter where you begin):

Hips

Medial and lateral rotations with respect to the age of the child:

- Lateral range is usually greater than medial range initially.
- Usually symmetrical by about 2 years of age.
- Be sure to test in hip extended and then flexed positions to check for soft tissue versus bony factors (Table 10.2)

Femur

Femoral torsion (twist within the shaft of the femur) should be reducing from birth. Clinically this can be assessed by a modified Ryder's test. This is a useful test to perform as it can clinically delineate the relative contributions of hip position and range from femoral torsion in children who display an intoeing gait.

Table 10.2 Examining hip ranges of motion

Infants and young children usually have greater lateral than medial hip range of motion, until age 2–3 years. From there on the hip range generally equalizes and the total range of motion reduces slightly with age. The clinician needs to be suspicious when the medial range exceeds the lateral and in particular if there is asymmetrical hip range of motion.

	Position	Structure
Ligaments	Lateral femoral position	Tight ischiofemoral ligament
	Medial femoral position	Tight pubofemoral ligament
		Tight iliofemoral ligament
Muscles	Lateral femoral position	Gluteus maximus
		Obturator externus
		Obturator internus
		Gemelli
		Quadratus femoris
		Piriformis
		Sartorius
		Adductor magnus
		Adductor longus
		Adductor brevis
	Medial femoral position	Iliopsoas
		Tensor fasciae latae
		Gluteus medius
		Gluteus minimus

Knee

Knee extension may be limited by:

- tight hamstrings
- tight proximal gastrocnemius
- tight ligaments.

Key Concepts

A typical compensation for reduced knee joint extension is adduction of the limb.

This is most noticeable when the child walks; as the forefoot loads, so the knee and hip begin to extend. If inadequate knee extension is available, adduction with heel lift will often be seen along with maintained knee flexion in some (more severe or neurological) cases.

Observe the position of the patella in both stance and gait (if walking). When the child stands facing you the patellae will normally be:

0–2 years: laterally rotated

>2 years: straight.

If the patellae are medially (or excessively laterally) rotated, there is at least some femoral component involved in the intoeing gait. If the patellae are straight but feet adducted, likely areas involved are:

- medial genicular rotation or bias (see Ch. 4)
- medial tibial torsion (see Ch. 4)
- metatarsus adductus (see Ch. 9)
- forefoot valgus/rigid plantarflexed first ray (see Ch. 4).

Tibia/fibular unit

Medial torsion According to Tachdjian (1985, 1997), medial tibial torsion is often associated with:

- metatarsus (adducto) varus
- genu varum
- tibial varum.

Remember that tibial torsion is minimal or absent at birth and then with neuromotor activity increases to 15–25° by approximately 8 years. True tibial torsion is difficult to measure and requires CT scans (usually not necessary). Clinically, malleolar position represents tibiofibular torsion and is 5° less (i.e. 10–20° lateral by 7–8 years).

Medial genicular position or bias According to Cusick (1990), genicular position can be typically medial in the young child as a consequence of initial intrauterine confinement. This should become symmetrical by approximately 3 years of age, but may be maintained if:

- severe initially
- postures perpetuate the position
- neuromotor dysfunction impedes normal modelling.

It is important to distinguish between medial genicular position (usually in children less than 3 years of age) and medial genicular bias, which is a lack of lateral genicular rotatory range and may need treatment in addition to changing aggravating sleeping or sitting postures.

Key *Concepts*

In gait, intoe due to medial tibial torsion is usually consistent whereas intoe due to medial genicular position tends to be more variable from step to step (Cusick 1990).

It is important to check tibiofibular rotations with hip extended and flexed to ascertain whether muscular contracture (hamstrings) is involved or if it is more statically ligamentous.

Feet

Metatarsus adductus is the most common foot condition that gives rise to an intoed gait pattern. There is association between metatarsus adductus and medial tibial torsion and also developmental dysplasia of the hip (Kumar & MacEwen 1982a, 1982b).

In an effort to function more abducted, a typical compensation at foot level in the intoed child is for the feet to excessively pronate. This reduces the adduction and looks better but at the possible expense of the feet later on. This compensation, which reduces adduction, may well be one of the reasons that intoe is often said to be 'outgrown' in time. Sometimes it is (e.g. reduction of medial genicular position), but at other times it causes a second alignment change which may improve cosmesis.

Muscle tone

Muscle tone is difficult to define (Illingworth 1987). It was previously thought that muscle tone was due to a constant 'background' neural activity, with high tone (hypertonus) indicating increased excitatory activity and low tone (hypotonus) the opposite. This concept has been disputed and tone is probably due to a combination of factors (e.g. reflex contraction, mechanical-elastic properties, such as stiffness, physical inertia) (Shepherd 1995).

As a result, the clinical assessment of muscle tone is based upon findings in a number of areas. The following factors are usually included in the assessment of muscle tone:

- observation of posture
- feel of the muscles
- resistance to passive motions
- range of motion
- reflex testing, e.g. tendon taps, plantar response, Moro and other anti-gravity responses (Illingworth 1987, Thomson 1993).

Muscle tone can and should be evaluated in several ways, taking into account each of the areas above. It takes experience to evaluate muscle tone and the clinician should always be checking for asymmetries of muscles groups, including strength and bulk.

Postures In very basic first impression terms, hypertonic children exhibit joint extension and consistently clenched fists, normal children show a flexed posture at rest and hypotonic children appear 'flat' against the resting surface.

Feel Hypotonic muscles feel softer and compress more easily when squeezed – they feel 'jellyish'. Hypertonic muscles feel as though they are contracted even though the child is relaxed – they feel more solid. Clearly it is easier to notice increased and reduced tone after experiencing the feel of normal muscle tone in children.

Resistance to passive motions For example modified Ashworth scale (Clopton et al 2005; Table 10.3). Excursion through passive joint range of motion and palpation of the muscle belly are probably the easiest.

Range of motion According to Illingworth, the most important lower limb joints to assess in an infant are the hip and the ankle (Illingworth 1987). Hip abduction and ankle dorsiflexion will be reduced in hypertonia and increased in hypotonia.

Joint hypermobility The Beighton scale is a useful clinical scoring system for assessing and rating generalized hypermobility in children (Table 10.4; van der Geissen et al 2001). A Beighton score of ≥5/9 is commonly used to define hypermobility. Hypermobility is generally:

Table 10.3 Modified Ashworth scale: a six-point scale to assess spasticity, resistance to passive muscle stretching

Grade	Description
0	No increased muscle tone
1	Slight increased muscle tone, showing as a catch and release/minimal resistance at end range of motion (ROM)
+1	Slight increase in muscle tone, showing as a catch followed by minimal resistance throughout remaining (<50%) ROM
2	More marked increase in muscle tone through most of ROM, but affected part still moves easily
3	Considerable increase in muscle tone, passive movement is difficult
4	Affected part is rigid in flexion or extension

In the lower limbs the common groups tested for children with spasticity are:
Hip adductors
Quadriceps
Hamstrings
Gastrocnemius
Soleus.

Table 10.4 Beighton scale (Fig. 10.1)

Assessment consists of the following (factors 1–4 score 0 or 1 for each area on both left and right sides; factor 5 score 0 or 1; the maximum total score is 9). The Beighton scale is clearly focused on the upper limb, hence the Lower Limb Assessment Score (LLAS) is pertinent for podiatrists (see Table 10.5).

Beighton scale assessment	Left	Right
1. Wrist flexion, e.g. thumb to forearm (Fig. 10.1A)		
2. Fifth metacarpo-phalangeal joint range, e.g. fifth finger extended to parallel forearm (Fig. 10.1B)		
3. Elbow hyperextension (Fig. 10.1C)		
4. Knee hyperextension (Fig. 10.1D)		
5. Lumbar flexion, e.g. can touch hands to floor with knees extended (Fig. 10.1E)		
Beighton scale total score –/9		

- more common in girls
- increased according to ethnicity (e.g. greater hypermobility in Asian children)
- often familial (a first-degree relative in approximately 2/3; Adib et al 2005)
- associated with joint pain, especially lower limb
- reduces with age.

Key *Concepts*

The Lower Limb Assessment Score (LLAS) better distinguishes children with hypermobility in the lower limbs and hence is more directly applicable for podiatrists (Table 10.5; Ferrari et al 2005).

The LLAS is reliable (inter-rater reliability assessed as 0.84 (ICC)). A LLAS score of 7/12 is the arbitrary cut-off score for hypermobility. It has been found that there is approximately 80% agreement between the LLAS and the Beighton scale, which indicates that children with lower limb hypermobility were also hypermobile in their upper limbs (Ferrari et al 2005).

It is important for the clinician to appreciate the possible overlap of children with joint hypermobility (JH) and genetic disorders such as Ehlers–Danlos syndrome (EDS), Marfan's syndrome and osteogenesis imperfecta (Adib et al 2005). EDS, Marfan's and osteogenesis imperfecta are associated with various musculoskeletal, eye and heart problems which need to be medically assessed.

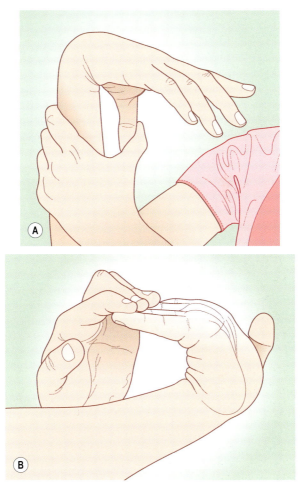

Figure 10.1 Beighton scale assessment (see Table 10.4).

Continued

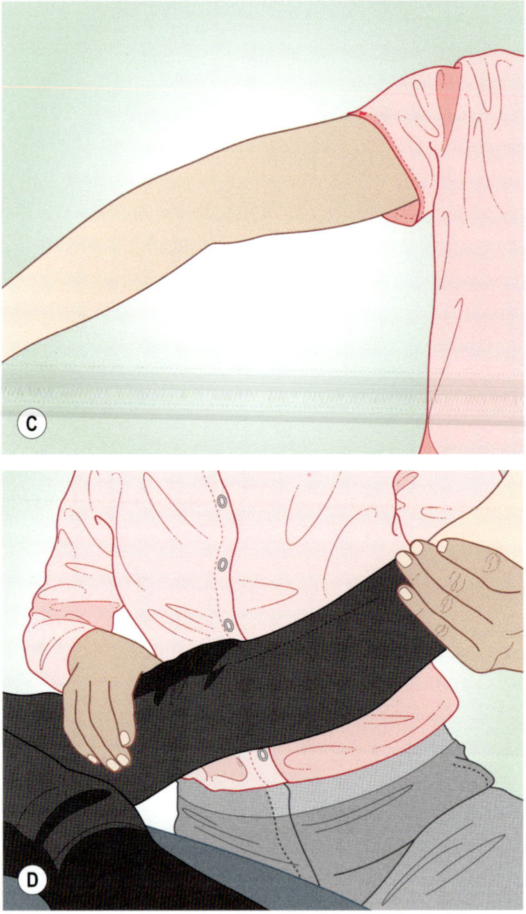

Figure 10.1 *Continued.*

JH may present as clumsiness, late walking and fine or gross motor skill difficulties. It is suggested that joint hypermobility may not be such a benign finding and that other organ systems may be involved, as indicated by the following observations in children with JH:

- increased rates of DDH and urinary tract infections (UTIs)
- boys with JH are constipated five times as often as controls

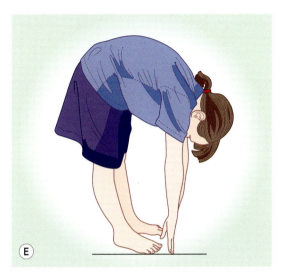

Figure 10.1 *Continued.*

- girls with JH are more prone to UTIs and urinary incontinence (Adib et al 2005).

Reflex testing The following reflexes are included in the lower limb and gait evaluation of children:

- ankle reflex (S1, 2)
- knee reflex (L3, 4)
- plantar response
- Chaddock's or Babinski's tests (Thomson 1993)
- plantar grasp response (Futagi et al 1999).

Key *Concepts*

See Chapter 5, Gait development.
   Differential diagnostic considerations for absent plantar grasp response or ankle reflexes.

Reflex testing provides an opportunity to evaluate the functional integrity of relatively small segments of the nervous system. As a result the findings are valuable in terms of both diagnosis and location of problems.

   Basically there are two types of reflexes: muscle stretch reflexes and cutaneous reflexes.

Table 10.5 Lower Limb Assessment Score (LLAS)

Tests 1–11 are performed with the child supine, test 12 is performed with the child standing. Each limb is scored separately and each 'yes' is given a score of 1. The total score is out of 12 (i.e. halve the total score for left and right, if symmetrical).

	Lower Limb Assessment Score (LLAS)	Left		Right	
	Examined criteria	Yes	No	Yes	No
1	Hip flexion • flex one hip, the other leg is extended • Does the thigh drop loosely to the chest with minimal force?				
2	Hip abduction • flexed hips, feet together, knees abduct to couch • Does lateral knee touch the couch with no/minimal force?				
3	Knee hyperextension • legs straight • Can heel be lifted ≥3 cm from couch with knee still touching?				
4	Knee anterior drawer test • hips, knees flexed, foot stabilized on couch • Does tibia move forward from femur? — moderate force, 'clunk' is a positive draw sign				
5	Knee rotation • hip, knee flexed, hold ankle at malleoli and rotate • Does tibial tubercle move ≥2 cm medial/lateral?				
6	Ankle dorsiflexion • knee flexed to 45°, firmly dorsiflex ankle • Does ankle dorsiflex ≥15°?				
7	Ankle anterior drawer test • knee flexed to 45°, firmly move heel forward • Do calcaneus/talus move anterior from tibia?				
8	Subtalar inversion • feet hang over end of couch, heel inverted on leg • Does sole of foot invert (visualized) 45° or more?				

Table 10.5 Lower Limb Assessment Score (LLAS) – cont'd

	Lower Limb Assessment Score (LLAS)	Left		Right	
	Examined criteria	Yes	No	Yes	No
9	Midtarsal inversion • feet hang over end of couch, forefoot held lateral-medial • Does forefoot invert (visualized) 45° or more?				
10	Midtarsal ab/adduction and dorsi/plantarflexion • feet hang over end of couch, heel stable, forefoot ab/d, d/pl • Does foot move >1 cm in any direction or 'wobble'?				
11	Metatarsophalangeal movement • feet hang over end of couch, hallux gently dorsiflexed • Does hallux dorsiflex >90°?				
12	Excessive subtalar joint pronation (weight-bearing) • child walks on spot, stops, inverts feet, relaxes • Does arch completely flatten, talus bulge medially? – end subtalar joint range should be reached				

Muscle stretch reflexes form the basis of normal neuromotor activity and so are very relevant to a child's gait patterns. Most commonly podiatrists test the:

- quadriceps reflex (*knee jerk*) L4
- Achilles reflex (*ankle jerk*) S1
- [hamstring reflex L4–S3]

Tendon taps need to be brisk, with the relevant tendon on slight stretch and the patient relaxed. Children are usually quite unsuspecting of reflex testing and hence good subjects. In older children who are wary and not relaxed, it may be necessary to *reinforce* the reflex loop by getting them to increase muscle activity elsewhere. Typically, the monkey grip is used, where the child links flexed fingers of their hands and pulls apart as instructed. Simultaneously, you tap the tendon to elicit the response.

Clinical *Tip*

> Placing the non-tapping hand on the anterior tibia (*knee jerk*) or plantar aspect of the foot (*ankle jerk*) will help the clinician to feel reflexive extension responses that are too 'soft' to see.
>
> A *reinforced* reflex response indicates an intact, if different, neural pathway. It is important to use the technique to avoid false impressions of absent reflexes, which are of great clinical concern.

Cutaneous reflexes are also normally occurring responses to stimuli, and are protective in nature. These responses are brief contractions of skeletal muscles following some form of noxious stimulus. Most commonly podiatrists test:

- plantar response: tibial nerve

Normal response to firm stroking across the plantar surface of the foot (using the sharp end of a reflex hammer tool from heel to lateral then medial metatarsal heads) is plantarflexion of the toes for 0.5 seconds. Abnormal response may include dorsiflexion of the hallux and splayed abduction of toes 2–5. This abnormal response is called the *Babinski response*. *Chaddock's* test is less noxious than Babinski's as it starts on the lateral side of the foot and then across the metatarsal heads and tests the same neural function.

Other factors

Muscle strength Muscle strength basically relates to the force a muscle can produce to either resist joint movement or to move a body part. Strength is determined by the number of motor units recruited for a particular task. The number of motor units recruited is related to the number of alpha motor neurons activated (Nolan 1996).

Muscle testing for grading strength of specific muscles is useful and should be used alongside a neurological and gait assessment. Strength testing means the examiner assesses the force of contraction a patient makes maximally and voluntarily. It is inherently subjective and only forms a part of the overall neuron-motor assessment (Shepherd 1995). Clearly a good working knowledge of the anatomy is crucial for muscle testing to be at all useful – i.e. origin, insertion, innervation, function.

For example, gastrocnemius:

- origin: femur
- insertion: tendo achilles
- innervation: tibial nerve, S1–S2
- function: plantarflexes the ankle.

Grading muscles is useful to assess both baseline status and progress over time, as shown in Table 10.7.

Weakness may be related to upper or lower motor neuron disorders, neuropathy or a more primary muscular dystrophy (e.g. Duchenne's; Gaudreault et al 2007). Muscle atrophy may coexist. Table 10.6 provides a summary of abnormal neurological patterns.

Sensation Sensory testing is performed in children in the usual manner, i.e. appreciating different nerve fibre types for testing and mapping the areas of loss or deficit as part of recording sensory deficit. Reference to dermatome mapping is helpful for specific nerve root distribution.

Vibration is a very useful perception to test as it addresses the smallest of the peripheral nerve fibres (type C) which have long been regarded as the hallmark for early sensory loss. A 128 Hz tuning fork provides the required frequency. A Rydel Seiffer tuning fork enables the frequency at which vibration perception is lost to be quantified.

The larger (type A) fibres detect painful stimuli, hence the traditional sharp/blunt discrimination which is now often replaced by the use of weighted monofilaments (normal subjects should detect a 1 gram monofilament while frankly neuropathic cases will not detect a 10 gram monofilament).

Thermal testing is theoretically ideal for testing the small peripheral fibres, but in practice cumbersome.

Light touch testing addresses the mechanoreceptors (type A fibres) and can be performed using a cotton wool ball or the traditional camel hair brush. *Allodynia* is the state of light touch being reported as painful (Nolan 1996).

Clearly any undetected injury (skin wound or abrasion from a splint or shoe) indicates significant sensory loss. It is important that the clinician

Table 10.6 Grading system for muscle strength

Description	Grade	%	Criteria
Normal	5	100	Full range of motion against gravity with maximum resistance
Good	4	75	Full range of motion against gravity with some resistance
Fair	3	50	Full range of motion against gravity only
Poor	2	25	Full range of motion with gravity eliminated
Trace	1	10	Palpable or visual sign of slight contraction without joint movement
Zero	0	0	No palpable or visual sign of muscle contraction

Table 10.7 Abnormal neurological patterns

Region of nervous system	Lower limb features	Other features
Cerebellar damage	Wide-based gait	Slurred speech, nystagmus
Upper motor neuron damage	Weak lower limb flexors, spasticity, hyperreflexia, extensor plantar response (Babinski, Chaddock)	Scissored gait with feet inverted and plantarflexed
Lower motor neuron damage	Muscle atrophy, hypotonia, weakness, areflexia, flexor plantar response	Fasciculations (spontaneous contraction of motor units)
Muscle disorders (e.g. Duchenne dystrophy, polymyositis)	Weakness and wasting of proximal limbs, normal sensation, normal reflexes	Swaggering gait, rolling motion of hips
Neuropathies	Distal loss of vibratory perception, reduced ankle jerks. Numbness, weakness may ensue	Foot drop may cause a steppage gait pattern

perform a thorough neuron-motor assessment and place the findings within the context of the child's entire presentation and clinical history.

Treatment

See Figure 10.2. If we understand the normal developmental trends of a child's angle of gait and apply some practical principles the decision as to when to employ treatment for a child with an intoeing gait becomes clearer.

Key Concepts

From the prevalence data presented earlier in this chapter, it seems likely that 10–30% of children up to 4–5 years of age may exhibit an intoeing gait pattern as a part of developmental variance.

Basic treatment options and indications are outlined below:

- Observe and monitor need for intervention (remember that the odds are for intoeing gait to reduce with age in the pre-school years and that few adults are seen to intoe).
- Change sitting and/or sleeping postures.
- Exercises as games (e.g. bear walks to stretch tight hamstrings).

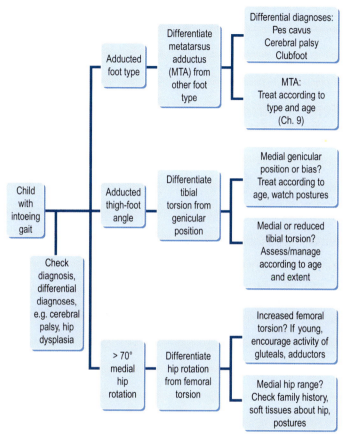

Figure 10.2 Algorithm for child with intoeing gait.

- Shoe selection (curved lasts and inflexible soles seem to increase an adducted gait).
- Serial casting–stretching.
- Gait plates (shown to reduce the adducted angle of gait by an average of 6° and to reduce tripping (Redmond 2000)).
- De-rotation splinting (seems to be effective for medial genicular bias with the added effect of changing sleeping postures, but not always very user friendly).

- In-shoe stabilizing (simple in-shoe wedging can reduce foot pronation, which in turn can reduce medial rotation of leg and knee).
- Surgery (for really problematic intoeing in children aged 10 or more years or in children with a neurological input such as cerebral palsy).

Treatment is justified if a child is repeatedly tripping and falling or if the condition is painful (unusual). Intoeing should be reducing with age, so extra attention and careful examination is warranted if intoeing is not reducing or is increasing with age.

Key Concepts

Asymmetry of the angle of gait should raise suspicion of a limb length difference, scoliosis or hemiplegia.

Evidence-based management

A systematic, evidence-directed approach to managing children with intoed gait is outlined in the algorithm shown as Figure 10.2.

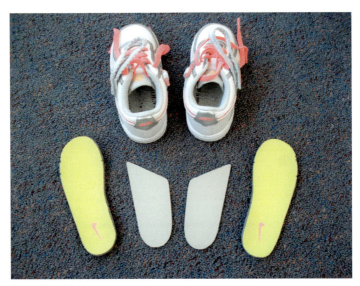

Figure 10.3 Gait plates.

Table 10.8

	Evidence hierarchy	Interventions
	Systematic review	None
	Randomized controlled trial	None
	Cohort	None
	Case control	None
	Case series	Gait plates
	Non-rating studies	Postures
		Shoes
		Torsion night splints
		Stretching
		Triplanar wedges

Children who trip and fall because of intoed gait patterns may be helped with the use of simple, inexpensive gait plates (Fig. 10.3). A tip for clinicians is to use shoes with a flexible forefoot to enhance abduction from heel lift to toe off.

Remember the basic steps to managing children with intoed gait are:

1. Be sure of the diagnosis – Table 10.1 will assist.
2. Use the best evidence available for management – see Figure 10.2, Table 10.8.
3. Monitor treatment outcomes – ask parents to record tripping or pain episodes.
4. Re-visit differential diagnoses and seek medical investigations if clinical picture changes from a regular intoeing presentation or definition.

References

Adib N, Davies K, Grahame R et al 2005 Joint hypermobility syndrome in childhood: a not so benign multisystem disorder? Rheumatology 44(6):744–750

Clopton N, Dutton J, Featherston T et al 2005 Interrater and intrarater reliability of the Modified Ashworth Scale in children with hypertonia. Pediatric Physical Therapy 17(4):268–274

Cusick BD 1990 Progressive casting and splinting for lower extermity deformities in children with neuromotor dysfunction. Therapy Skill Builders, Arizona

Fabry G, Cheng LX, Molenaers G 1994 Normal and abnormal torsional development in children. Clinical Orthopaedics and Related Research (302):22–26

Ferrari J, Parslow C, Lim E et al 2005 Joint hypermobility: the use of a new assessment tool to measure lower limb hypermobility. Clinical and Experimental Rheumatology 23(3):413–420

Fixsen JA, Valman HB 1981 Minor orthopaedic problems in children. BMJ 283:715–717

Futagi Y, Suzuki Y, Goto M 1999 Clinical significance of plantar grasp response in infants. Pediatric Neurology 20(2):111–115

Gaudreault N, Gravel D, Nadeau S et al 2007 A method to evaluate contractures effects during the gait of children with Duchenne dystrophy. Clinical Orthopaedics and Related Research (45):51–57

Ho CS, Lin CJ, Chou YL et al 2000 Foot progression angle and ankle joint complex in preschool children. Clinical Biomechanics 15:271–277

Illingworth RS 1987 The development of the infant and young child: normal and abnormal, 9th edn. Churchill Livingstone, London

Katz K, Wielunsky E, Krikler R et al 1991 Effect of neonatal posture on later lower limb rotation and gait in premature infants. Journal of Pediatric Orthopedics 11(4):520–522

Kumar SJ, MacEwen GD 1982a Torsional abnormalities in children's lower extremities. Orthopedic Clinics of North America 13(3):629–639

Kumar SJ, MacEwen GD 1982b The incidence of hip dysplasia with metatarsus adductus. Clinical Orthopaedics and Related Research (164):234–235

Li YH, Leong JCY 1999 Intoeing gait in children. Hong Kong Medical Journal 5(4):360–366

Lincoln TL, Suen PW 2003 Common rotational variations in children. Journal of the American Academy of Orthopaedic Surgeons 11(5):312–320

Losel S, Burgess-Milliron MJ, Micheli LJ et al 1996 A simplified technique for determining foot progression angle in children 4 to 16 years of age. Journal of Pediatric Orthopedics 16(5):570–574

Morcuende JA, Ponseti IV 1996 Congenital metatarsus adductus in early human fetal development. Clinical Orthopaedics and Related Research (333):261–266

Morcuende JA, Dolan LA, Dietz FR 2004 Radical reduction in the rate of extensive corrective surgery for clubfoot using the Ponseti method. Pediatrics 113(2):376–380

Nolan MF 1996 Introduction to neurologic examination. FA Davis, Philadelphia

Redmond AC 2000 The effectiveness of gait plates in controlling in-toeing symptoms in young children. Journal of the American Podiatric Medical Association 90(2):70

Rethlefsen SA, Healy BS, Wren TAL et al 2006 Causes of intoeing gait in children with cerebral palsy. Journal of Bone and Joint Surgery – American Volume 88(10):2175–2180

Ryan DJ 2001 Intoeing: a developmental norm. Orthopaedic Nursing 20(2):13–18

Sass P, Hassan G 2003 Lower extremity abnormalities in children. American Family Physician 68(3):461–468

Shepherd RB 1995 Physiotherapy in paediatrics, 3rd edn. Butterworth Heinemann, Oxford

Song HR, Choonia AT, Hong SJ et al 2006 Rotational profile of the lower extremity in achondroplasia: computed tomographic examination of 25 patients. Skeletal Radiology 35(12):929–934

Svenningsen S, Terjesen T, Auflem M 1990 Hip rotation and in-toeing gait: a study of normal subjects from four years until adult age. Clinical Orthopaedics and Related Research (251):177–182

Tachdjian MO 1985 The child's foot. WB Saunders, Philadelphia

Tachdjian MO 1997 Clinical pediatric orthopedics. Appleton and Lange, Stamford, CT

Tervo RC, Azuma S, Stout J et al 2002 Correlation between physical functioning and gait measures in children with cerebral palsy. Developmental Medicine and Child Neurology 44:185–190

Thackeray C, Beeson P 1996a In-toeing gait in children: a review of the literature. The Foot 6:1–4

Thackeray C, Beeson P 1996b Is in-toeing gait a developmental stage? The Foot 6:19–24

Thomson P 1993 Introduction to podopaediatrics. WB Saunders, London

Valmassy RL 1996 Clinical biomechanics of the lower extremities. Mosby, St Louis, p. 246

van der Geissen LJ, Liekens D 2001 Validation of Beighton score and prevalence of connective tissue signs in 773 Dutch children. Journal of Rheumatology 28(12):2726–2730

Wenger DR, Leach J 1986 Foot deformities in infants and children. Pediatric Clinics of North America 33(6):1411–1427

Weseley MS, Barenfeld PA, Eisenstein AL 1981 Thoughts on in-toeing and out-toeing: twenty years' experience with over 5000 cases and a review of the literature. Foot and Ankle 2(1):49–57

Widhe T 1997 Foot deformities at birth: a longitudinal prospective study over a 16-year period. Journal of Pediatric Orthopedics 17:20–24

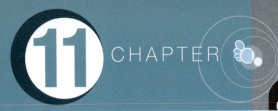

Toe walking

Definition

A gait pattern in which heel contact with the ground is excluded, either completely or periodically, Toe walking may be idiopathic (i.e. of unknown cause), developmental or associated with a particular condition.

Introduction

Toe walking is the broad term used to describe the gait pattern in children who walk without making ground contact with their heels. Toe walking can be a developmental phase in young children or it may indicate an underlying pathology. Differentiation between normal or *idiopathic* toe walking and more serious entities is at the core of assessment of affected children.

Key *Concepts*

Toe walking is a common gait variant and considered normal in children under 2–3 years (Armand et al 2006, Hemo et al 2006, Kogan & Smith 2001, Stricker & Angulo 1998). Most children will have a consistent heel-to-toe pattern by the age of 2 years (Stricker & Angulo 1998).

Aetiology

The cause of idiopathic toe walking (ITW) is largely unknown but a family history is attributed in 30–71% of cases (Eiff & Steiner 2006). An increased number of type 1 muscle fibres in gastrocnemius bellies have been implicated histologically (Stricker & Angulo 1998).

Prevalence

The incidence in the general population is not known, but has been estimated to occur in 7–24% of normal children (Sobel et al 1997).

Key *Concepts*

The key issue when dealing with a child presenting as a toe walker is to determine whether the presentation is idiopathic or associated with specific pathology, especially cerebral palsy or muscular dystrophy.

Diagnosis

This distinction is the nub of diagnosis and future treatment considerations.

Checklist for children with cerebral palsy

- Spasticity, brisk reflexes.
- Premature term birth history.
- Low birth weight.
- Late motor milestones.
- Knee flexion at heel strike.

Checklist for children with muscular dystrophy

- Falls increase with age.
- Get up from floor in a climbing pattern (Gower's sign; Sutherland et al 1981).
- Extensor weakness (Gaudreault et al 2007).
- Reduced ankle dorsiflexion.

Classification

Idiopathic toe walking (ITW) has recently been classified based on a gait analysis severity scale (Alvarez et al 2007). The classification system utilizes the ankle rocker model (Perry et al 2003) to delineate three sub-types of ITW (Table 11.1, Fig. 11.1). Foot slap indicates inadequate extensor function to the control the first rocker. Lack of sagittal plane ankle range disturbs the second rocker and is commonly indicated by an early lift of

Table 11.1 Idiopathic toe walking type as defined by kinematic and kinetic observations Diagnosis of ITW type directs the clinician's decisions about treatment of these children.

ITW/ analysis	Kinematic	Kinematic	Kinetic	Clinical	
Type	First rocker present	Early third rocker present	Predominant first ankle plantarflexion moment	Ankle range dorsiflexion	Treatment indicated
1 Mild	Yes	No	No	Normal	No
2 Moderate	Yes or no	Yes or no	No	Normal or reduced	No, review
3 Severe	No	Yes	Yes	Reduced or negative	Yes

ITW = idiopathic toe walking.

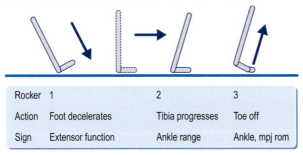

Rocker	1	2	3
Action	Foot decelerates	Tibia progresses	Toe off
Sign	Extensor function	Ankle range	Ankle, mpj rom

Figure 11.1 Diagrammatic representation of the ankle rocker model.

the heel, flattening of the foot and increased angle of foot abduction. The third rocker requires timed firing of the triceps surae to achieve ankle plantarflexion and forward propulsion. There must also be a stable and adequate range of motion available at the first metatarsophalangeal joint. Gait was assessed to visualize three main criteria:

Type 1 Mild

Presence of the first ankle rocker (kinematic):

- normally occurs from heel strike to maximum ankle plantarflexion with loading in the first 12% of the gait cycle
- present if initial ankle angle is greater than 5° plantarflexion.

Type 2 Moderate

Presence of an early third ankle rocker (kinematic):

- normally occurs after 40% gait cycle when ankle plantarflexion ends heel contact at the completion of the second rocker phase
- present if third rocker occurs before or at 30% of the gait cycle.

Type 3 Severe

Predominant first ankle moment (kinetic):

- compares the initial stance ankle plantarflexion moment with the peak ankle plantarflexion moment of late stance
- present if the first ankle plantarflexion moment is greater than the second ankle plantarflexion moment, indicative of increasing ankle plantarflexion in early stance (Fig. 11.1).

Using this classification system in a study of the gait patterns of 133 children (266 feet) with ITW (average age 8 years), the following type proportions were found:

Type 1 (mild)	40 feet
Type 2 (moderate)	129 feet
Type 3 (severe)	90 feet

(Seven feet were unable to be classified; Alvarez et al 2007).

Differential diagnosis

Cerebral palsy, muscular dystrophy, clubfoot deformity, autism, short Achilles tendon and neuropathy have all been associated with toe walking gait patterns (Armand et al 2006, Hemo et al 2006, Hirsch & Wagner 2004). *Idiopathic* toe walking (ITW) is diagnosed by excluding other under-lying pathologies and remains the term used to describe a toe–toe gait pattern (Armand et al 2006, Kogan & Smith 2001). Children with ITW typically walk on their toes but are usually able to make heel contact when requested.

It can be especially difficult to distinguish ITW from diplegia (Kogan & Smith 2001, Policy et al 2001, Sobel et al 1997). However, children with ITW usually have normal milestones for walking in comparison to children with diplegia, who begin to walk later (Kogan & Smith 2001). In addition, children with ITW display maximum knee extension at heel contact as opposed to children with cerebral palsy who have a flexed knee at heel strike (Eiff & Steiner 2006).

Typical clinical picture

Parents usually present with concern about their child's toe walking after the age of 3 years, when very few other children exhibit this gait pattern and when it becomes constant rather than transient. There may be peer pressure issues when children are at school. Teachers, grandparents, friends and neighbours may also comment on the child's gait. Toe walking may be seen as cute 'twinkle-toes' in little children, but can become a source of embarrassment and grounds for teasing in older children.

History and examination

Predisposing factors may include:

- family history of ITW
- premature birth
- male gender.

Differential diagnosis includes:

- cerebral palsy
- autism
- muscular dystrophy
- sensory integration problems, e.g. tactile defensiveness
- developmental delay
- triceps surae contracture or shortness.

Clinical findings

The first goal of the clinician is to discern whether the child presents with ITW or toe walking due to another aetiology, with main concerns being cerebral palsy and muscular dystrophy. Other differential factors must also be considered.

Subsequently, the clinician then focuses more on the gait pattern and the available ankle range of motion. Observation of stance and gait will quickly reveal whether the child can weight-bear on their heels and whether they can consciously walk with an instigated heel strike (Fig. 11.2). It is also useful to see if these children can squat with either heel-to-toe weight-bearing or just forefoot-toe weight-bearing – or not at all. This usually informs the hands-on physical examination.

Ankle range needs to be examined with the knee in both extended and flexed positions to isolate soleus from gastrocnemius.

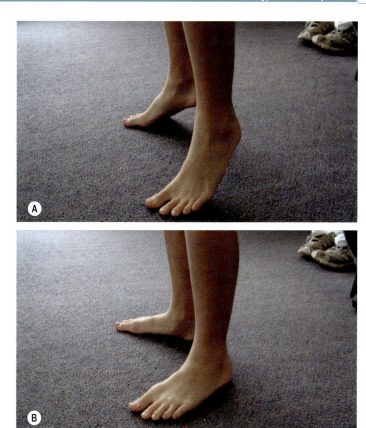

Figure 11.2 (A) It is important to establish if children who ITW can stand plantigrade. (B) The foot will often be pronated and flattened as compensation, especially in type 3 ITW.

Key Concepts

The available range of ankle dorsiflexion is variable in normal children but should be available to some extent. ITW types 1 and 2 will have ankle dorsiflexion available. Those with type 3 ITW will have very reduced or no ankle dorsiflexion available (Table 11.1, Fig. 11.3).

The concept of first and second resistances for testing joint range can be usefully applied (see Ch. 4).

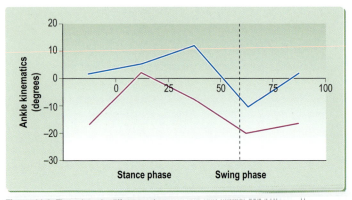

Figure 11.0 The gait cycle differences between TTW and normal gait patterns. The kinematic absence of ankle dorsiflexion should match the clinically observed reduced range of motion. Discovering which timings of the gait cycle are most aberrant enhances the clinical management of these children by being able to specify the structures and functions which most impede the gait from being normal.

Medical findings and considerations

As podiatrists, we are not able to diagnose the more global neuromotor diseases which may be present in children who present with a toe walking gait pattern. However, we should be aware of abnormal signs and liaise with paediatricians for full diagnosis and management.

Some factors to be alert to include:

- Reflex testing: usually normal, can be brisker than usual (check for spasticity, i.e. ankle clonus, early 'catch' with knee extension, e.g. Tardieu scale). A paediatrician and paediatric physiotherapist should be consulted.

- Response to touch: tactile defensive children may incorporate toe walking into their motor patterns in an effort to reduce surface contact area and hence noxious sensory stimuli from the feet. These children will generally have associated signs, e.g. non-crawlers but 'bottom-scufflers', wriggle and squirm when dressed or dried after a bath, difficult to feed, dislike being held or cuddled, always want clean hands. These children can benefit from an occupational therapy assessment and sensory desensitization programme.

- Unilateral toe walking: suspect hemiplegia or talipes equinovarus (clubfoot) primarily.

- Onset of falling: an increase in falling over as a child gets older can be indicative of Duchenne muscular dystrophy (affects boys only) or other muscular, neurological problems. Have the child get up from the floor to test for Gower's sign, where the child is seen to struggle and 'climb' up their own legs to stand (pathognomonic for Duchenne muscular dystrophy; Gaudreault et al 2007, Sutherland et al 1981).
- Calf hypertrophy: check the parents' calf group bulk for size and ankle joint range. In conjunction with a history of ITW, there may well be familial factors.

Clinical Tip

Children who always sleep prone tend to have reduced ankle dorsiflexion. This seems especially the case with ITW but can also be an aggravating factor for calcaneal apophysitis (Sever's), Achilles tendinopathy and heel pain sufferers.

Associations

ITW has been associated with premature birth (<37 weeks' gestation), developmental delay, male gender, autism and positive family history (Stricker & Angulo 1998).

Treatment

Classification of toe walking according to severity based type will help to direct the treatment planning for children exhibiting ITW (Alvarez et al 2007). Treatment options basically divide into conservative versus surgical options (see Table 11.2):

Conservative

- stretching
- night splints
- serial casting
- Botulinum toxin type A (Botox®) injections.

Surgical

- tendo Achillis (TA) lengthening (postoperative casting).

Table 11.2 The available research for managing toe walking positioned on the hierarchy of evidence

The best current evidence for management of ITW is for either:

- intramuscular botulinum toxin type A (Botox®) injection and casting the leg in knee extension and maximum ankle dorsiflexion
- surgical lengthening of the Achilles tendon.

Evidence hierarchy	Interventions
Systematic review	None
Randomized controlled trial	None
Cohort	Achilles tendon lengthening Botox® + casting
Case control	Stretching Serial casting
Case series	Serial casting Achilles lengthening
Non-rating studies	Splinting

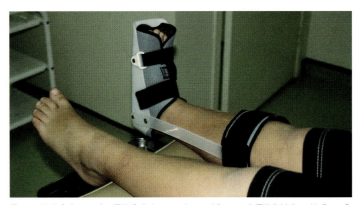

Figure 11.4 Splint use for ITW. Splinting may be used for type 3 ITW (initially, with Botox® or postoperatively). Type 2 ITW may also benefit from splint use, especially if ankle range reduces clinically as may happen after a growth spurt.

Evidence-based management (Table 11.2)

The best current evidence for management of ITW is for either:

- intramuscular Botox® injection and casting the leg in knee extension and maximum ankle dorsiflexion
- surgical lengthening of the Achilles tendon.

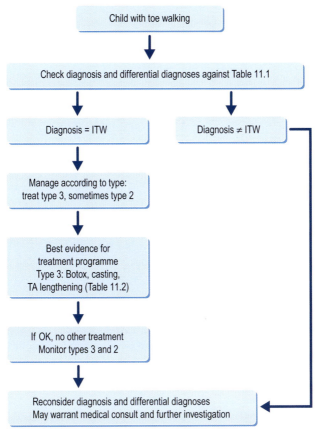

Figure 11.5 Algorithm for diagnosis, classification and treatment of ITW.

The evidence for management of ITW has been largely anecdotal and opinion-based rather than tested science (Babb & Carlson 2008).

Key *Concepts*

Classification of idiopathic toe walking by type helps to direct treatment.

In general only type 3 ITW requires treatment as it displays poor ankle range passively and in gait, abnormal ankle rocker formation and abnormal ankle kinetics (Alvarez et al 2007).

Casting, splinting and stretching protocols have not been shown to be successful. Incomplete correction and recurrence are frequent findings (Stricker & Angulo 1998). Surgery has shown some improved outcomes, but complications have been associated (Stricker & Angulo 1998). The use of Botox® has been shown to improve ITW gait and is used in conjunction with casting/splinting/stretching (Fig. 11.4) and perhaps Achilles tendon lengthening in older children who exhibit type 3 ITW (Alvarez et al 2007, Brunt et al 2004).

The basic steps to managing children with toe walking are outlined in Figure 11.5 and include:

1. Be sure of the diagnosis – exclude cerebral palsy, muscular dystrophy and other possible causes.

2. Use the best evidence available for management:

   a. type 0 ITW should be treated

   b. type 2 should be monitored

   c. type 1 should not be treated.

3. Monitor treatment outcomes – for types 3 and 2.

4. Re-visit differential diagnoses and seek medical investigations if the clinical picture changes from ITW.

References

Alvarez C, De Vera M, Beauchamp R et al 2007 Classification of idiopathic toe walking based on gait analysis: development and application of the ITW severity classification. Gait and Posture 26:428–435

Armand S, Watelain E, Mercier M et al 2006 Identification and classification of toe-walkers based on ankle kinematics, using a data mining method. Gait and Posture 23:240–248

Babb A, Carlson WO 2008 Idiopathic toe-walking. South Dakota Medicine 61(2):53–57

Brunt D, Woo R, Kim H 2004 Effect of botulinum toxin type A on gait of children who are idiopathic toe-walkers. Journal of Surgical Orthopaedic Advances 13:149–155

Eiff MP, Steiner E 2006 What is the appropriate evaluation and treatment of children who are 'toe walkers'? Journal of Family Practice 55(5):1–3

Gaudreault N, Gravel D, Nadeau S et al 2007 A method to evaluate contractures effects during the gait of children with Duchenne dystrophy. Clinical Orthopaedics and Related Research (45):51–57

Hemo Y, Macdessi SJ, Pierce RA et al 2006 Outcome of patients after Achilles tendon lengthening for treatment of idiopathic toe walking. Journal of Pediatric Orthopedics 26(3):336–340

Hirsch G, Wagner B 2004 The natural history of idiopathic toe-walking: a long-term follow-up of fourteen conservatively treated children. Acta Paediatrica 93:196–199

Kogan M, Smith J 2001 Simplified approach to idiopathic toe-walking. Journal of Pediatric Orthopedics 21:790–791

Perry J, Burnfield JM, Gronley JK et al 2003 Toe walking: muscular demands at the ankle and knee. Archives of Physical Medicine and Rehabilitation 2003; 84:7–16

Policy JF, Torburn L, Rinsky LA et al 2001 Electromyographic test to differentiate mild diplegic cerebral palsy and idiopathic toe-walking. Journal of Pediatric Orthopedics 21:784–789

Sobel E, Caselli MA, Velez Z 1997 Effect of persistent toe walking on ankle equinus. Journal of the American Podiatric Medical Association 87(1):17–22

Stricker SJ, Angulo JC 1998 Idiopathic toe walking: a comparison of treatment methods. Journal of Pediatric Orthopedics 18(3):289–293

Sutherland DH, Olshen R, Cooper L et al 1981 The pathomechanics of gait in Duchenne muscular dystrophy. Developmental Medicine and Child Neurology 23(1):3–22

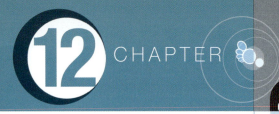

Verrucae

Introduction

Warts or *verrucae* are a frequently occurring dermatological problem in children (and to a lesser extent, adults). These benign, highly vascular neoplasms affect the plantar surface of the foot as well as other skin surfaces of the feet (also hands and elsewhere). As podiatrists are frequently consulted about these lesions it is important that diagnosis and management be accurate and effective. It is also important that the podiatrist provides good and current information as the *'plantar wart'* may still conjure potent notions of fear and dread.

Diagnosis

Unlike the raised dome shape of the common wart, plantar warts (by definition located on the sole or plantar surface of the feet) are flattened due to the weight-bearing loads which push them into the skin's dermis (Fig. 12.1; Bryant et al 2003).

Plantar warts are often indistinct in initial appearance as there is usually overlying callus. Upon debridement of the overlying callus there are often black spots in the middle of a circumscribed lesion, caused by capillary thrombosis (Gawkrodger 2003). A verruca can grow to half an inch in diameter and may spread into a cluster of small warts, often termed a *mosaic* wart.

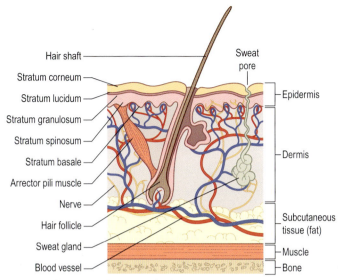

Figure 12.1 Skin structure in cross-section view.

The diagnosis of plantar warts is usually obvious, although they are sometimes confused with corns (heloma dura) or an embedded foreign body. It is very easy to differentiate warts by checking the following clinical signs (Fig. 12.2):

- *The 'squeeze test'*: gently squeezing the sides towards the centre of a wart will be painful; not so with a corn; usually not so with a 'splinter' (unless already infected).
- *Skin line parallels*: callus debridement of a wart reveals deviated epidermal ridging (rete ridges) around a wart; the lines remain parallel with a corn or foreign body.
- *Location*: a wart will not necessarily be adjacent to bone; a typical corn (by definition) will always be adjacent to bone.

If it is not a corn or a splinter, is it definitely a wart?

Usually, but not always, so it is important to include the following differential diagnoses (Gawkrodger 2003, Jennings et al 2006, Young & Cohen 2005):

- amelanotic melanoma
- fibroma
- molluscum contagiosum (pox virus)

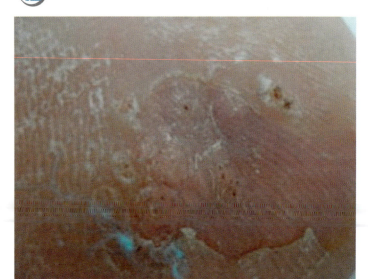

Figure 12.2 Multiple verrucae on the heel of a 14-year-old girl. Note the interruption of epidermal ridge parallels and thrombosed capillaries.

- skin cancer (solar keratosis)
- pyogenic granuloma
- arsenical keratosis
- lichen planus
- squamous cell carcinoma
- basal cell carcinoma
- epidermoid cyst
- xanthoma.

Key *Concepts*

If the appearance is not typical, definitive diagnosis of questionable lesions should be obtained by skin biopsy (Jennings et al 2006, Levy & Hetherington 1990).

Aetiology

Warts (verrucae) on the feet are caused by the human papilloma virus (HPV) of which there are some 80 different types identified (Gibbs & Harvey 2006). HPV types 1, 2 and 4 are specifically associated, although type 2 is more commonly associated with lesions on the hands rather than the feet (Gawkrodger 2003). HPV incubation time ranges from 4 weeks to 20 months (Jennings et al 2006). HPV is very contagious, but can only be transmitted by direct contact. Infection on the plantar aspect of the foot usually occurs through a small loss of skin integrity as in cuts, fissures and abrasions. HPV thrives in warm, moist environments such as footwear, swimming pools, changing room floors and bathrooms. If an infected bare foot walks across the poolside, there may be a release of virus-infected cells onto the floor. Other people can pick the virus up, especially if small cuts and abrasions are present on their feet which promote the virus's penetration to become a parasite within the keratino-cytes (Levy & Hetherington 1990). Warts tend to be common in children, especially teenagers, where they can seem to reach almost epidemic proportions. However, for unknown reasons, some people seem to be more susceptible to the virus while others are immune (similar to the herpes simplex virus which causes *cold sores*).

Verrucae usually disappear in time when the host immune system mounts an adequate response, and thus the general policy or clinical wisdom is to only treat warts which are:

- causing pain
- located on the plantar aspect of the feet.

Most verrucae generally resolve spontaneously within 6 months in healthy children, but in adults they can persist for years. It is cited that 50–66% resolve within 2 years (Gibbs et al 2002, 2006; Kilkenny & Marks 1996; Paller 1996; Young & Cohen 2005).

Prevalence

There have been estimates that some 7–10% of the population may be affected by warts on their feet (Jennings et al 2006). The prevalence has been found to increase with children's age, with warts (not only plantar) found in 12% of children aged 4–6 years and 24% of 16–18-year-olds (Kilkenny et al 1998).

Typical clinical picture

Classically the child presents with the following story from their parents: their child has been complaining of sore foot and thinks there may be something embedded in it. The site will often determine the level of dis-comfort, which tends to increase if weight-bearing and as the lesion grows.

When taking the case history of children with verrucae, it is clearly vital that the clinician is familiar with the inclusion/exclusion criteria and appre-ciative of the concerns raised. Some children and their parents are quite anxious and need to be both informed and reassured. Helpful information may include:

- Positively identifying the lesion – wart vs corn vs splinter vs other.
- Explaining and demonstrating how you have diagnosed a wart (e.g. deviated skin striations, positive 'squeeze' test).
- Informing the patient/parent that a wart is a common viral skin infection in children and that on average ⅔ resolve within 2 years.
- Explaining what a 'plantar' wart is and why treatment is often indicated.
- Explaining the best evidence treatment vs many treatment myths.
- Outlining the treatment programme, i.e. frequency of visits, experience of treatment, treatment duration estimate.
- Advising about contagious contact for home care, e.g. shared bathrooms, avoiding bare feet.

Evidence-based management (Table 12.1)

Historically, there has been a veritable plethora of cited ways to treat verrucae. Everything from rubbing the wart with cow dung or an old wash cloth to 'selling' the wart and many other options, lotions and potions have been expounded and recommended (Tax 1980, Young & Cohen 2005). The immunological response to the HPV means that warts often resolve spontaneously, yet this can be an event that latently coincides with some form of treatment, rendering the uninitiated patient or clinician confident in the intervention used. Many treatment modes have been employed indicating that none are uniformly effective as most are not directly anti-viral (Parsad et al 1999).

Key Concepts

Cell mediated immunity (CMI) is generally regarded as the main mechanism for wart regression.

Specific titers of IgM have been detected in patients actively infected, while IgG has been found in patients with regressing warts (Jennings et al 2006). Various immunotherapies have been used to treat warts, including cimetidine, ranitidine and levamisole which are thought to inhibit suppressor T-cell function by blocking type 2 histamine receptors (Mullen et al 2005, Paller 1996, Parsad et al 1999). Despite eager initial support from low-quality studies (Paller 1996, Parsad et al 1999), better trials (Yilmaz et al 1996) and a recent systematic search (Fit & Williams 2007) have not

Table 12.1

Salicylic acid preparations have the best evidence for treatment of warts, being supported by a Cochrane Library systematic review. This should be the clinician's first-line treatment.

Evidence hierarchy	Interventions
Systematic review	Salicylic acid
Randomized controlled trial	Salicylic acid
	Cryotherapy
	Intralesional bleomycin
	Fluorouracil
	Intralesional interferons
	Dinitrochlorobenzene
	Photodynamic therapy
	Pulsed dye laser
Cohort	Cimetidine
	Levamisole
Case control	None
Case series	Cimetidine
	Glutaraldehyde
	Formaldehyde
	Podophyllin
	Cantharidin
	Surgery (curettage and excision)
Non-rating studies	

supported histamine 2 antagonists (e.g. cimetidine, ranitidine) for the treatment of warts.

Table 12.1 illustrates interventions and the respective positioning on the evidence hierarchy model (Sackett et al 2000).

Key Concepts

> Clearly the best evidence and thus the first-line approach for management of verrucae is topical salicylic acid.

A systematic review of the literature has supported topical preparations containing salicylic acid for over 5 years (Gibbs & Harvey 2006, Gibbs et al 2002). In summary, systematic review of the literature has found:

- Topical Salicylic acid has been found to be effective and more effective than placebo (73 vs 48%).

- Average cure rate of placebo preparations was 27%.
- Evidence for cryotherapy was surprisingly lacking. Cryotherapy has been found to be no more effective than salicylic acid or duct tape occlusion.

Economic treatment costs

Following on from the systematic review, which advocates preparations incorporating salicylic acid, the economic costs of the most commonly used wart treatments have been assessed. The costs of over-the-counter (OTC) salicylic acid preparations were compared with cryotherapy from a GP and found to be almost half the cost. OTC duct tape was costed at $\frac{1}{3}$ of salicylic acid, which warrants further investigation in terms of effectiveness (Koogh Brown et al 2008, Thomas et al 2006).

Psychosocial considerations

Despite the fact that warts are common skin infections and an acknowledged bane for both patients and clinicians, very little has been written about the morbidity of warts on children's feet. Quality of life (QoL) data have now found that common feelings are:

- Embarrassed by warts (81%).
- Fear negative comment from others (70%).
- Frustrated by persistence of warts (90%).
- Frustrated by recurrence of warts (69%) (Ciconte et al 2003).
- Moderate to extreme discomfort (51%).
- Affected social or leisure time (38%).

Warts on the feet are more associated with discomfort and less associated with fear of a negative comment from others (being hidden in comparison to lesions on hands; Ciconte et al 2003).

Key *Concepts*

Up to 30% of patients with skin problems suffer psychological distress (Gawkrodger 2003).

It is useful for clinicians to acknowledge these emotions when dealing with children and parents of children with warts.

Remember the basic steps to managing children with verrucae are:

1. Be sure of the diagnosis:
   - should be obvious; check differential diagnoses if not and consider another opinion and a skin biopsy.

2. Assess the wart:
   – duration (remember that $\frac{1}{2}$ to $\frac{2}{3}$ resolve in 2 years)
   – pain
   – location
   – size, type.
3. Use the best evidence available for management (Table 12.1)
4. Monitor treatment outcomes – measure size of wart.
5. Re-visit differential diagnoses and seek medical investigations if clinical picture changes:
   – skin biopsy is the 'gold standard'.
6. If the child is immunosuppressed, adapt expectations to be realistic.
7. Outline the treatment plan options and expectations, explaining the variable response of the virus.

Treating children with *EASE*

This simple acronym illustrates a useful approach to take when treating children for nearly all conditions (and adults too, for that matter). It has evolved from my years as a clinician treating children and is underpinned by the observation that children are very cooperative if they understand why treatment is needed, what is going to happen, if it will hurt and if they can stop it. I tell children if a treatment will hurt and ask them to help by telling me how they are coping as we progress. I use language such as the following (age adjusted) prior to debriding a wart:

We have to scrape off the dead skin so that the paint/cream gets closer to the wart to kill it faster. Otherwise the paint has to eat through all of the dead skin before it even reaches the wart. I'll be as gentle as I can with the scraping, it usually feels a bit scratchy. It might be a bit uncomfortable, but you'll be OK. Tell me if it bothers you, I promise I'll stop if you say so, but I do need you to keep still while I'm doing it. It won't take long.

I have children lying down and don't make the scalpel obvious. Often a book can distract them and enlisting the help of parents can be needed for hand-holding and reassurance if the child is frightened.

EASE explained

*E*xplain
   Talk first – but not too much detail and not for too long – get on with it (more time often equals more time to wind up fear)

*A*ttitude

Physical: lie them down; make them comfortable with a pillow, book, parent

Mental: be positive, perceptive, but also matter-of-fact as the job has to be done

*S*cience: the first and second line approach

1. First line: best evidence for first-line approach is salicylic acid (Gibbs & Harvey 2006)

Dry for 48 hours

Repeat 10–14 days

[but watch the literature for trials investigating low-cost duct tape]

2. Second line: cryotherapy (Keogh-Brown et al 2008)

*E*valuate

Treatment outcomes:

monitor lesion size, child's pain, child's activity

Cost/benefit for child:

Costs:

- pain of treatment
- frequency of visits
- economic costs to family

Benefits:

- eradicating a painful wart
- alleviating painful weight-bearing.

References

Bryant B, Knights K, Salerno E 2003 Pharmacology for health professionals. Mosby, Sydney

Ciconte A, Campbell J, Tabrizi S et al 2003 Warts are not merely blemishes on the skin: a study on the morbidity associated with having viral cutaneous warts. Australasian Journal of Dermatology 44:169–173

Fit KE, Williams PC 2007 Use of histamine2-antagonists for the treatment of verruca vulgaris. Annals of Pharmacotherapy 41(7):1222–1226

Gawkrodger DJ 2003 Dermatology: an illustrated colour text, 3rd edn. Churchill Livingstone, Oxford

Gibbs S, Harvey I 2006 Topical treatments for cutaneous warts. Cochrane Database of Systematic Reviews 2006:(3): Art.No.: CD001781

Gibbs S, Harvey I, Sterling JC et al 2002 Local treatments for cutaneous warts: systematic review. BMJ 325:1–8

Gibbs S, Harvey I, Sterling JC et al 2006 Local treatments for cutaneous warts. Cochrane Database of Systematic Reviews 2006:(2)

Jennings MB, Ricketti J, Guadara J et al 2006 Treatment for simple plantar verrucae: monochloroacetic acid and 10% formaldehyde versus 10% formaldehyde alone. Journal of the American Podiatric Medical Association 96(1):53–58

Keogh-Brown MR, Fordham RJ, Thomas KS et al 2008 To freeze or not to freeze: a cost-effectiveness analysis of wart treatment. British Journal of Dermatology 156(4):687–692

Kilkenny M, Marks R 1996 The descriptive epidemiology of warts in the community. Australasian Journal of Dermatology 37(2): 80–86

Kilkenny M, Merlin K, Young R et al 1998 The prevalence of common skin conditions in Australian school children: 1. Common, plane and plantar viral warts. British Journal of Dermatology 138(5):840–845

Levy LA, Hetherington VJ 1990 Principles and practice of podiatric medicine. Churchill Livingstone, New York

Mullen B, Guiliana JV, Nesheiwat F 2005 Cimetidine as a first-line therapy for pedal verruca. Journal of the American Podiatric Medical Association 95(3):229–234

Paller AS 1996 Cimetidine for the treatment of warts. Western Journal of Medicine 164(6):520–521

Parsad D, Saini R, Negi KS 1999 Comparison of combination of cimetidine and levamisole with cimetidine alone in the treatment of recalcitrant warts. Australasian Journal of Dermatology 40:93–95

Sackett DL, Straus SE, Richardson WS et al 2000 Evidence-based medicine: how to practice and teach EBM, 2nd edn. Churchill Livingstone, London

Tax HR 1980 Podopediatrics. Williams and Wilkins, Baltimore, p. 52

Thomas KS, Keogh-Brown MR, Chalmers JR et al 2006 Effectiveness and cost-effectiveness of salicylic acid and cryotherapy for cutaneous warts: an economic decision model. Health Technology Assessment 10(25):iii, ix–87

Yilmaz E, Alpsoy E, Basaran E 1996 Cimetidine therapy for warts: a placebo-controlled, double-blind study. Journal of the American Academy of Dermatology 34(6):1005–1007

Young S, Cohen GE 2005 Treatment of verruca plantaris with a combination of topical fluorouracil and salicylic acid. Journal of the American Podiatric Medical Association 95(4):366–369

Further reading

Bryant B, Knights K, Salerno E 2003 Pharmacology for health professionals. Mosby, Sydney

Gawkrodger DJ 2002 Dermatology: an illustrated colour text, 3rd edn. Churchill Livingstone, London

Sport and the osteochondroses

Definition

The term osteochondroses is used to describe a group of distinct conditions, affecting children between the ages of 2 and 16 years, which involve the growth plates of developing bones. Some of these conditions can severely limit the young athlete.

> **Key** Concepts
>
> Depending upon the anatomical site and the extent of the condition, effects of the osteochondroses can be either transient or chronic.

Introduction

The child sports participant presents a range of unique issues to the clinician. Some three-quarters of all sports injuries in children have been found to involve the lower limb. The practitioner needs to have good knowledge of developmental biomechanics, sports played and also injury management to be able to diagnose and manage these children effectively.

Children's unique and susceptible developmental features are outlined below (Brukner & Khan 1993, Frank et al 2007). Each of the following factors play a part:

Osseous growth precedes soft tissue growth

This often results in functional inflexibility and reduced joint ranges of motion until soft tissue elongation occurs. Coordination may be affected as running styles adapt to a changing musculoskeletal frame.

Growth 'spurts' increase injury risk

Puberty is associated with twice the usual injury incidence rate. Skeletal growth in parallel with increased sporting participation and intensity can see the young sportsperson side-lined with injury which diminishes both participation and enjoyment.

Apophyses

The apophyses are growth plates (epiphyses) with tendinous attachment which are susceptible to traction forces as muscle–tendon units contract. By definition the apophyses are transient within osseous development, but significant lower limb sites can be a focus of apophyseal inflammation, pain and functional restriction, e.g. tibial tubercle (Osgood–Schlatter's), calcaneus (Sever's).

Epiphyseal activity

Like the apophyses, the very existence of these growth centres delineates children's skeletons from those of adults where the epiphyseal activity has ceased. These regions are more vulnerable to injury and if the growth plate per se is involved, it may retard the final development of that region.

Peer/gender inequality

As Figure 13.1 illustrates, females and males develop at different rates and there is also variable development within same gender age groups. Differing body mass and strength can be implicated in injury outcomes, an obvious example being injuries from collision where disparate body masses are involved.

Injury mechanisms

There are basically two types of injuries that occur in children playing sports: *macrotrauma* or *microtrauma*. Macrotrauma is usually due to collision in comparison to microtrauma, which is an overuse injury of the child's body – too much activity and too frequently played.

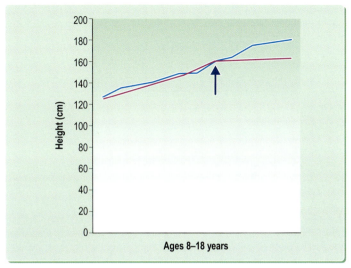

Figure 13.1 Growth as measured by height/age by gender. From age 13 years, boys and girls growth deviates markedly. During secondary school sports, boys' growth is far more active than girls' growth, which has injury implications.

Less common but more serious differential diagnoses need to be considered and may include:

- epiphyseal growth plate injury
- greenstick fractures
- stress fractures
- bone tumours.

Stress–strain curve

A strain on a material can be defined by the change in the material's dimension, and any force acting on a material produces a stress (y). With tensile materials, strain (x) is the same as stretch, and is simply the ratio of the change in size to the original size. *Young's modulus of elasticity* (E) is the ratio between stress and strain:

$$E = y/x$$

E is the slope of the stress–strain graph: the steeper the slope, the stiffer the material. The maximum height of the stress–strain curve is called the tensile strength, which is a measure of the amount of stress a material can take before tearing apart. The extensibility, or breaking strain, is the furthest horizontal extent of the stress–strain curve and, like strain, it is dimensionless. We can graph Young's modulus to see how stiffness changes as strain increases.

Young's modulus of elasticity can be thought of as a measure of how well a substance stands up to tension.

Let us consider the concepts offered by Young's modulus in relation to the young athlete:

The ligaments in children are relatively stronger than the adjacent bone or cartilage. As a result the young athlete often incurs bone or epiphyseal fracture when the same injury in an adult would produce ligament disruption, e.g. lateral ankle inversion sprain. The child is much more elastic than the adult.

The muscle–tendon unit, which is commonly injured following excessive strain in adults, is usually spared in children, who are more likely to develop pathology at the tendon–bone junction, e.g. Sever's (calcaneal apophysis) versus Achilles tendon problems. Tendon ruptures are very unusual in the young athlete.

The child's bony skeleton, like the tendons and ligaments, shows a vast ability to absorb load without major damage. Young bone is more pliable than older more brittle bone. However, young bone will often injure before young soft tissues, especially if bone is loaded repetitively (giving inadequate repair time) or if a huge load is applied (i.e. macrotrauma) (Ch. 3).

Key *Points*

- The child is much more elastic than the adult.
- Tendon ruptures are very unusual in the young athlete.
- Young bone is more pliable than older more brittle bone.
- Young bone will often injure before young soft tissues.

Bone mineral density

Total body calcium advances from 25 grams at birth to 1000 grams by 15–20 years. Low bone mass results in increased fracture risk, with the aetiology of osteoporosis being multifactorial. Fracture risk may be due to the failure to reach peak bone mass (poor nutrition and low physical activity in childhood are common factors) or accelerated bone loss (smoking, alcohol, reduced exercise, poor diet). Both genetic and environmental factors influence bone mass. Maternal hip fracture history doubles the risk of hip fracture in white women (Seeman 1996). Lean body mass, alcohol intake, cigarette smoking, lack of exercise and diet depleted in calcium, phosphorus, vitamins A, B_{12}, C, D are all implicated factors.

Adult influences

The 'ugly' adult who barracks loudly from the sidelines and urges children to 'win!, win!' does not realize that their child is unlikely to have winning as their primary concern when they participate in sport. Numerous authors (Brukner & Khan 1993, Frank et al 2007, Gould 1990) have found a mismatching of desired outcomes between children playing sports and the adults around them (parents, coaches, trainers). It has been found that coaches' and parents' excessive desire to win (through their children) actually reduces children's enjoyment of sport and promotes the 'drop-out' rate (Brukner & Khan 1993, Dyment 1991).

It is pertinent to look at the reasons children play sport. It has been found that most young athletes are motivated to play because they want to have fun and enjoy the games. Winning is much lower on their priority list. The drop-out rate of children from sport has been found to be very much influenced by the adult's *'win, win'* bias. There are enormous implications for the health dollar if children are inadvertently discouraged from sports and physical activity.

Recent data have estimated that on average Australians are gaining weight at a rate greater than 1 gram per day. Overweight, obesity, diabetes, metabolic syndrome and mental illness may all be reduced by maintaining regular exercise and physical fitness. Regular exercise is an important part of developing a healthy lifestyle and it is recommended that young people are physically active for 60 minutes each day (Sports Medicine Australia 2008).

Preventing sports injuries in children: basic principles
Proactive: injury prevention

- Encouraging children to play a range of sports not only reduces injuries from physical overuse but also builds better overall skills.
- Warm up and cool down as part of training and playing are recommended.
- Levels of training need to be age appropriate. Sports Medicine Australia provides *Safety Guidelines for Children in Sport* (www.sma.

org.au; readers should investigate comparable guidelines in their own countries).

- Hydration, weather, diet, sun protection and footwear are all important and changing needs for children playing sport.
- A school or sporting club pre-participation musculoskeletal screening of children is very useful to detect children who are at increased injury risk. Flexibility, posture, biomechanics, motor skills are areas which can be assessed such that children can better avoid potential injuries (www.smartplay.com.au).

Reactive: injury management

- RICER (**r**est, **i**ce, **c**ompression, **e**levation, **r**eferral).
- No HARM (no **h**eat, no **a**lcohol, no **r**unning, no **m**assage).
- It is often necessary to reduce training loads by up to 50% in the acute stages. It is important to be aware how distressing this can be for young sports participants and it is beneficial to spend time explaining the costs and benefits. It is often possible for sport to continue if loads are reduced.
- Local measures to accommodate injuries can be effective in maintaining sport participation (e.g. heel raises for Sever's cases).
- Correcting identified faults is an essential part of injury management, prevention and better ongoing performance. Typically, areas which need to be addressed include:

Muscular imbalances, e.g.:
- hamstrings and quadriceps
- triceps surae and long foot extensors
- peroneals and tibialis posterior.

Faulty biomechanics:
- supinated/cavus feet (prone to ankle inversion injury)
- pronated feet (prone to MTSS, PFS; see page 261).

- Reviewing young athletes is important, especially pre-season. Footwear advice is fundamental to this process as the wrong choice can be problematic in terms of injury and expensive to correct.

Specific lower limb problems

The osteochondroses are an interesting group of conditions which affect the developing skeleton, making active children susceptible.

Key *Concepts*

Lower limb osteochondroses are dominated by Osgood–Schlatter's disease (affecting the knee/tibial tubercle), which is the most common, and Perthes' (*Legg–Calvé–Perthes'*) disease (affecting the hip), which is potentially the most consequential.

While often transient (e.g. Sever's, affecting the heel), the osteochondroses are important as they can prevent or deter children from sport. Subsequent implications, such as reduced physical activity, can be far reaching when we consider the rise of childhood obesity. Although often referred to as '*diseases*', the osteochondroses are finite conditions and many do not have lasting sequelae (there are notable exceptions in some cases of Perthes', Freiberg's and Köhler's). These conditions are largely specific to children, involving growth plates, which are eliminated with epiphyseal closures (Bloomfield et al 1992, Brukner & Khan 1993, Gould 1990).

The osteochondroses are a group of conditions affecting the growth plates. Although the aetiology of the osteochondroses is not particularly well understood, the non-articular types are associated with overuse. A possible interplay between mechanical and vascular factors may occur, where increased forces may diminish bone blood flow and in turn the less perfused/weaker bone yields more easily to loads.

Classification

An ordered classification is a useful guide for the clinician dealing with any of the osteochondroses (Bloomfield et al 1992). Table 13.1 uses this approach for the conditions to be discussed within this chapter.

The most commonly encountered osteochondroses (lower limb vicinity) are discussed in the following sections. Table 13.2 provides a useful clinical summary.

Spine

Scheuermann's disease

Osteochondrosis results in kyphosis of the spine, especially in the thoracic or thoracolumbar regions. This may be complicated by a compensatory and increased lumbar lordosis. A physiotherapy or orthopaedic opinion should be sought.

Radiological findings confirm diagnosis, with wedging of three or more vertebrae at 5° or greater angulation (lateral view). Management generally

Table 13.1 Classification of the osteochondroses*

	Non-articular	Articular		Physeal
		Crushing, subchondral	Splitting, chondral	
Scheuermann's				X
Legg-Calvé-Perthes'		X		
Slipped capital epiphysis**				
Osgood–Schlatter's	X			
Sinding–Larsen–Johansson	X			
Sever's	X			
Iselin's	X			
Freiberg's		X		
Köhler's		X		
Buschke's		X		
Osteochondritis dissecans			X	

*Each condition can be classified as non-articular, articular or physeal.
**Really a Salter–Harris type 1 fracture or epiphysiolysis.

consists of stretching, strengthening exercises and sometimes bracing is indicated. Once kyphosis reaches 50° or more, surgery is usually considered necessary (Scuderi & McCann 2005).

Hip

Slipped capital epiphysis

Avascular necrosis of the epiphysis classically occurring in 12–15-year-old males who present with a limp. It is usually bilateral.

Orthopaedic management, which is aimed at containing the head of femur within the acetabulum, consists of rest, selecting appropriate sports, surgery as needed (internal pin fixation).

This condition, while often included in the discussion of osteochondroses, is really a *Salter–Harris type I* fracture (Ch. 3). It generally occurs in active, overweight boys aged 12–15 years who have grown rapidly. The contralateral hip is involved in at least 25% of cases and a limp is typical (Myers & Thompson 1997). Treatment consists of rest, open reduction and internal fixation of the epiphysis. The risk is avascular necrosis of the femoral head.

Table 13.2 Summary of the common lower limb (or associated) osteochondroses

While uncommon, the differential diagnosis of a bone tumour must always be included in the clinician's differential diagnostic work-up.

	Age (years)	Structure	Factors	Onset	Differential diagnoses
Scheuermann's	12–16	Thoracic spine	Increased thoracic kyphosis and lumbar lordosis Sports: gymnastics Tight hamstrings	**a.** painful **b.** non-painful – typical	Scoliosis Disc disease
Legg–Calvé–Perthes'	4–10	Femoral head	More common in boys	Limp, refuse to weight-bear	Femoral head necrosis
Slipped capital epiphysis	12–16	Femoral head	More common in boys	Growth spurts	Fracture of physis
Osgood–Schlatter's	8–15	Anterior tibial tubercle	Patella alta Imbalance between hamstrings and quadriceps	Kicking sports Running Jumping	Osteogenic sarcoma
Sinding–Larsen–Johansson	8–15	Inferior patella pole			
Sever's	8–15	Calcaneal apophysis	Tight triceps surae Poor footwear Growth Poor training Pronated foot	Heel pain Limp Worse barefoot Worse in morning Pain with 'squeeze'	Brodie's abscess Osteomyelitis Sero-negative status

Continued

Table 13.2 Summary of the common lower limb (or associated) osteochondroses—cont'd

	Age (years)	Structure	Factors	Onset	Differential diagnoses
Iselin's	8–15	5th metatarsal styloid process	Poor footwear Growth Pronated foot	Lateral foot pain Limp Shoes aggravate Local tenderness Worse with forefoot abduction	Os vesalianum Peroneus brevis Lateral plantar fascial slip Apophyseal fracture
Freiberg's	12–16	2nd metatarsal head (or 3rd, 4th)	Foot type Sports Shoes Training	Local tenderness Dorsal prominence Reduced MPJ range	Stress fracture
Köhler's	2–8	Navicular	Spontaneous Pronated foot Pre-coalition	Limp Non-weight-bearing Local tenderness	Osteomyelitis Sero-negative status Tumour
Buschke's	4–6	Cuneiforms	Rare, not known	Limp	Fracture

MPJ = metatarsophalangeal joint.

Legg–Calvé–Perthes' disease

An articular subchondral osteochondrosis of the femoral head, which is usually unilateral, causing a limp, and occurring in children aged between 4 and 10 years. Boys are affected four times more than girls and (gender related) reduced bone age may be associated. Characterized by aseptic necrosis, subchondral fracture, revascularization, and repair of bone.

Key Concepts

Clinically there will be reduced or guarded hip abduction of the affected side (Fig. 13.2).

Diagnostic tests include X-rays, ultrasound scans, blood tests. Initial synovitis has been reported as has increased proteoglycan fragments. An increase in stromelysin 1 has been associated with poor prognosis and earlier osteoarthritis (Eckerwall et al 1997). Management usually includes rest, range of motion exercises and sometimes a brace.

Knee

Osgood–Schlatter's disease

Osgood–Schlatter's disease, an apophysitis, is the most frequently occurring osteochondrosis in the lower limb and has the potential to be very

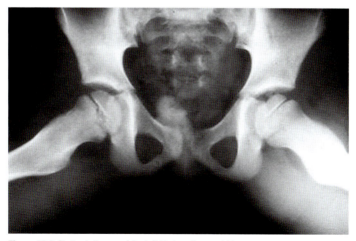

Figure 13.2 Perthes' disease of the left hip in a 7-year-old boy.

disabling for the young athlete. It may also be referred to as osteochondritis or epiphysitis of the tibial tuberosity and patellar (quadriceps) tendon junction. The patellar tendon itself may also be injured, as occurs in the so-called 'jumper's knee'. Osgood–Schlatter's disease involves avulsion of forming tibial tubercle by sudden or protracted contractions of the body's largest muscle force, the quadriceps complex.

Osgood–Schlatter's usually occurs in 12–15 year olds and is characterized by a very tender and often effused tibial tubercle.

Key Points

The differential diagnoses which must be noted are:

- Osteochondrosis of the femoral condyle (local effusion)
- Osteogenic sarcoma (10–30 years)
- Sinding–Larsen–Johansson (see below).

The management of Osgood–Schlatter's will depend on how acute the initial clinical presentation is and what level of activity the child occupies (Fig. 13.3). Overall the approach consists of:

- RICER.
- Stretching – especially hamstrings, gastrocnemius, quadriceps.
- Biomechanics – foot posture may affect tibial rotation and knee position.
- Modify training – reduce sport by 50% until symptoms are adequately alleviated.

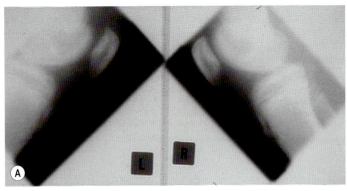

Figure 13.3 (A) Osgood–Schlatter's disease of the right knee. The disruption of the tibial tubercle was more marked than the left side and was clinically inflamed and tender.

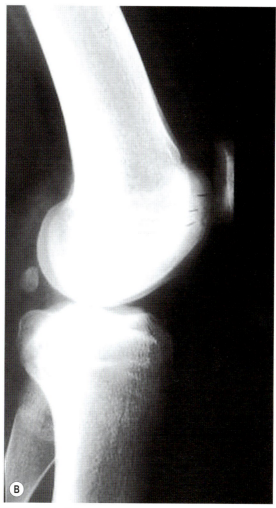

Figure 13.3 *Continued.* (B) Patella alta in Osgood–Schlatter's disease in a 14-year-old runner.

Additional factors which are relevant and need to be considered are:

Patella alta The patella is positioned proximally relative to the femoral condyles which strains the patellar tendon at its tibial attachment, aggravating the tibial apophysis. Tight quadriceps and hip flexors may be associated (Aparaicio et al 1997).

Lateral tibial torsion May be a predisposing mechanical factor for the onset of Osgood–Schlatter's, as for many knee disorders. A CT study found that subjects with Osgood–Schlatter's disease had some 16° greater lateral tibial torsion when compared with control subjects (Gigante et al 2003).

Increased disability by age 20 years It has been reported that subjects with a history of Osgood–Schlatter's score lower on scales assessing both activities of daily living and sports activity than subjects without this same history (Ross & Villard 2003).

Patellar tendon attaches more proximally and broadly to tibia An MRI study has indicated that subjects affected with Osgood–Schlatter's disease have altered attachment between the patellar tendon and tibia compared with unaffected subjects (Demirag et al 2004).

Sinding–Larsen–Johansson (SLJ)

Sinding–Larsen–Johansson (SLJ) is osteochondritis of the inferior patella pole (Brukner & Khan 1993).

SLJ is less common and poorly recognized in comparison to Osgood–Schlatter's, even though it is anatomically only a few centimetres away, attached to the superior end of the patellar tendon. Presentation of localized anterior knee pain in the young sporting participant should include careful palpation of:

• inferior patellar pole:	Sinding–Larsen–Johansson
• patellar tendon:	patellar tendinopathy
• anterior tibial tubercle:	Osgood–Schlatter's

Further consideration should be given to the complex of patellofemoral syndrome (PFS) so that other anatomical structures are also included in the clinical examination:

- hamstrings: range of motion (medial vs lateral); straight leg raise (neural component)
- menisci: flexed compression, McMurray's test
- cruciate ligaments: anterior/posterior drawer, Lachmann's test
- collateral ligaments: flexed distraction
- cursae: subpatellar (Brukner & Khan 1993).

Tibia

Osteochondritis

The main ('true') osteochondroses involve the knee and patellofemoral region as stated above. There are also many other lower limb conditions which need to be taken into account when examining the young sports enthusiast.

- 'Shin splints' or medial tibial stress syndrome (MTSS). Classically this presents in the track and field athlete, who exhibits imbalance between lower limb flexors (especially tibialis anterior, extensor digitorum longus) and extensors (triceps surae, principally gastrocnemius, although it is important not to overlook soleus – the soleal fascia – which has also been implicated).
- Stress fracture. In effect this is a progression of unrelenting MTSS and/or compartment syndrome where the periostitis gives way to periosteal elevation (classic X-ray sign) and cortical disruption of the diaphyseal shaft (Fig. 13.4).
- Compartment syndrome.

Key Concepts

The bellies of the ankle flexors in athletes and dancers may develop elevated intra-compartmental pressure if the muscle hypertrophies beyond the range of the myofascial extensibility.

This is why the classic presentation of compartment syndrome is a pain that comes on during activity and increases in parallel with exercise (pressure rising) to halt the athlete but falls away quickly once activity ceases (pressure drops). (In contrast MTSS pain comes on during exercise, can be 'run through' but is still symptomatic when activity stops.) Young dancers and gymnasts are typically implicated.

- Posterior tibialis dysfunction. Posterior tibial tendinopathy results from inflammation of the tendon or sheath and is often due to chronic excessive pronation. This places excessive tension at the insertion point onto the navicular, which may already be prominent or have an associated supernumerary projection. Need to differentiate from an avulsion fracture of the tendon (especially if there is a lot of effusion and pain), periostitis, os tibiale externum.

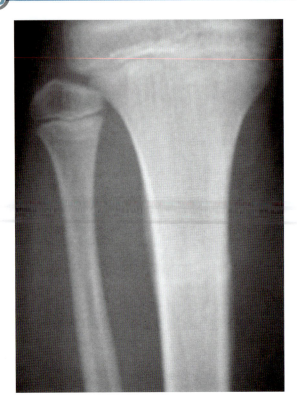

Figure 13.4 Tibial stress fracture in an 11-year-old boy. Note the periosteal elevation of the medial tibial cortex. This boy had 24-hour pain and a concerning differential diagnosis was an osteogenic sarcoma (eliminated by these films).

Further differential diagnoses include:

- Still's disease, part of the seronegative spectrum.
- Blount's disease (Accadbled et al 2003), associated with increased genu varum.
- Osteochondritis dissecans, fragmentation and possible separation of the epiphysis. Subchondral bone appears primarily affected, with secondary effects on articular cartilage, which may separate to 'catch' within the knee joint as young sufferers will frequently describe. Imaging for diagnosis, rest and/or surgery may be required (Crawford & Safran 2006).

Ankle

Ankle equinus is the lack of adequate sagittal plane dorsiflexion and can usually be assessed as one of four basic types:

1. gastrocnemius

2. soleus

3. gastroc/soleal

4. osseous (e.g. anterior tibial exostosis) (Chs 4, 5, 11).

Assessment

Lie the child prone and assess ankle range by observing the angle between the lateral border of the foot and the lateral leg (approximating the fibula) when the foot is dorsiflexed. Approximately 5–10° of ankle dorsiflexion should be seen. Less than 5–10° dorsiflexion, with the knee extended, is a *gastrocnemius equinus* (the most usual). If the dorsiflexion range is also limited when the knee is flexed this is a *gastroc-soleal equinus*. If the ankle dorsiflexion is reduced with the knee flexed but not when the knee is extended, this is a *soleal equinus*. If the ankle dorsiflexion range is reduced in both knee extended and flexed positions and there is a sudden or 'hard' quality to the end of range, suspect an *osseous equinus* (can confirm with plain lateral X-ray).

It is really useful to test muscle range with the first and second resistance approach (used primarily, but not exclusively, for children with increased neuromotor tone; Tardieu et al 1988), as described in Chapter 4. Using this method the concept of first (R1) and second resistance (R2) levels of muscle testing are given to reflect the functional muscle length (R1) versus the connective tissue capability (R2). Clinically it is accepted that R2 – R1 is the range to be gained from muscle stretching whereas a deficit in R2 may indicate the need for pharmaceutical (Galli et al 2001) or surgical interventions (Saraph et al 2001).

Equinus may be functional or fixed depending upon the aetiology involved. Children with cerebral palsy often exhibit an overtly destructive lack of ankle dorsiflexion which results in deforming forces in the foot skeleton in the transverse (foot abducts) and frontal/coronal (foot everts) planes. These compensations are seen in non-neurological cases too, but the forces, and hence the skeletal deformity, are less. Left unchecked, equinus participates in a biomechanical cascade which may potentiate a flat foot, hallux valgus and altered gait. A 'bouncy' walk is typical. Reduction in the contact phase of gait means that both the midstance and propulsive phases are also affected. The net result is poor foot position and efficient musculoskeletal leverage. In short, gait becomes compensated and multiple problems may arise (Chs 4 and 11).

Inversion sprains

Ankle inversion sprains are a debilitating injury for any athlete and with young children may involve avulsion of the fibular epiphysis rather than just ligament damage which occurs with the same injury mechanism in adults.

Key Concepts

The lateral ankle ligaments are generally injured in the order of anterior talofibular ligament (ATFL) (common), calcaneofibular ligament (CFL) (less common), posterior talofibular ligament (PTFL) (really nasty and unlucky)

There are multiple stages to recovery, including the initial diagnosis of structures involved (watch the sural nerve), RICER approach and an assessment of risk factors prior to returning to sport. The use of braces after ankle injury is supported by research, whereas the use of high-top footwear and wobble boards is equivocal, although often favoured by convention (Handoll et al 2001).

Rear foot

Sever's disease

Calcaneal apophysitis is the most common of the osteochondroses seen in children's feet. A traction apophysitis of tendo Achilles/calcaneal junction, Sever's occurs most usually between the ages of 8 and 14 years. It is thought to be due to excessive impact forces as well as traction and is often associated with ankle equinus and pronated foot posture (Evans 2001a).

Clinically, the picture includes a child of susceptible age, often with a limp on the affected side/s (or a reported limp after sports), ankle equinus and a positive response to squeezing the heel. These children often have poor footwear (lack of, or negative, heel height), poor training practices (no warm-up or cool-down regimen) and may be subject to physical overuse (school, club and social sports). Rapid increase in musculoskeletal growth is often associated with functional inflexibility and sometimes reduced physical coordination is noticed.

First described by Dr J.W. Sever in 1912, Sever's '*disease*' is a clinical diagnosis with no specific X-ray findings (Evans 2001a). Radiologically, there may or may not be visible epiphyseal fragmentation, which can also occur without symptomatic apophysitis, so radiological findings are not pathognomonic (Fig. 13.5).

Management generally consists of the RICER approach, stretching triceps surae, checking/changing shoes, foot biomechanics, e.g. heel raises for sport, orthoses if indicated (often not required and hence should not be dispensed routinely). The need to modify sport participation

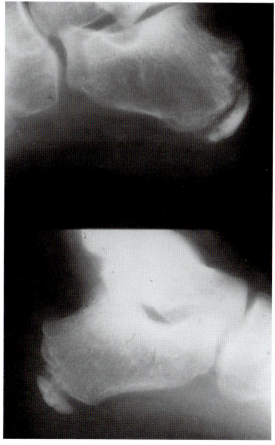

Figure 13.5 Sever's disease. Radiological findings are not definitive, so the diagnosis remains clinical. Marked sclerosis and fragmentation of the epiphysis are also seen in asymptomatic children. This X-ray is diagnostically inconsequential.

and practices is a crucial area to address, as it is often a primary contributor. The child and the parents need to be well supplied with information so that they understand the vulnerability of growth plate sites, but that the aim of treatment is to continue sports involvement, not to negate it.

Differential diagnoses should include:

- osteomyelitis (usually effusion and inflammation is visible)
- rheumatoid arthritis
- calcaneal fracture
- tumour, e.g. Brodie's abscess
- neural tension (Evans 2001b).

If Sever's disease is unresponsive to usual treatments (uncharacteristic), the possibility of a metaphyseal fracture should be considered (Ogden et al 2004). This is usually not the case.

Whilst Sever's is the most usual rear foot problem to present in the sporting child, other entities need to be appreciated and understood as well.

Tarsal coalition

Coalitions (joining of bones) may affect:

- calcaneus and navicular
- calcaneus and cuboid
- talus and calcaneus
- talus and navicular (Fig. 13.6).

These children usually present with foot pain and a limp. There is usually an easily discernible reduction in subtalar joint range of motion. A plain X-ray may show the coalition if osseous (a *synostosis*), but most symptomatic coalitions are cartilaginous (a *synchondrosis*). A fibrous coalition (a *syndesmosis*) may or may not be symptomatic. CT or MRI are the preferred imaging modalities, especially if surgery is being considered. Some coalitions respond very well to conservative management (shoes, orthoses) but many require surgery.

Os trigonum

This ossicle occurs in approximately 10–15% of the population (Sarrafian 1993) and functionally limits ankle joint plantarflexion. It is most problematic in dancers, particularly if *en pointe* position is attempted in ballet. Gymnasts and martial arts participants are also hindered and describe an acute, sharp pain with rapid ankle plantarflexion. An os trigonum is easily visible on a plain lateral X-ray and may need to be surgically excised to restore ankle range and relieve symptoms.

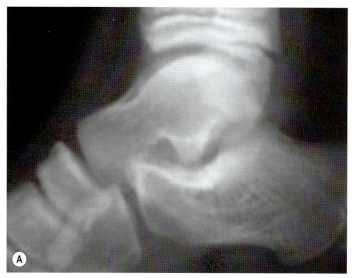

Figure 13.6 (A) Symptomatic coalition of the talo-calcaneal joint in a 14-year-old boy as seen on X-ray. Cast immobilization was used for ambulating until surgical correction was convenient (for schooling).

Achilles tendinopathy

This is not a common finding in children, but can occur in sprinters especially if ankle dorsiflexion is limited. In older children/young adults the Alfredson programme may supplement the usual management approach of ice, lunge calf stretches and extensor group strengthening (Alfredson & Cook 2007).

Clinical Tip

Sever's, Achilles problems and toe walking can be helped by eradicating a prone sleeping posture (also benefits adults with heel pain, e.g. 'plantar fasciitis').

Midfoot

Navicular

Being the last foot bone to ossify (variably between 3 and 5 years; Evans et al 2003), the navicular can be a vulnerable bone in the young child. The specific osteochondrosis of the navicular is Köhler's disease. First

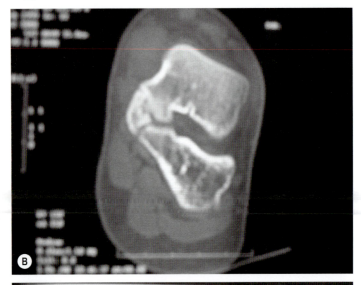

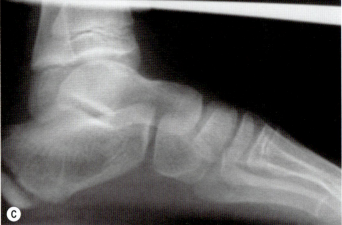

Figure 13.6 *Continued.* (B) Symptomatic coalition of the talo-calcaneal joint in a 14-year-old boy as seen on CT.
(C) An asymptomatic tarsal coalition of the talo-navicular joint in a 13-year-old schoolboy. The affected right foot is two sizes smaller than the unaffected left foot. There is no appreciable limb length difference and this boy is very active (football, cricket, swimming).

described by Dr Köhler in 1908, this condition will cause a limp or refusal to weight-bear in affected children. Köhler's disease may affect children as young as 2 years of age. The upper age limit is approximately 8 years of age and males are predisposed at least fourfold.

Sonography is often the best imaging modality in children less than 5 years of age, as the navicular may not be sufficiently ossified to show clearly with X-rays (this varies).

Key Concepts

Avascularity of the navicular is the main concern with Köhler's disease.

Once diagnosed, treatment initially consists of a weight-bearing below-knee cast for 6 weeks. Supportive footwear and high-flanged foot orthoses may be required to reduce tension from the posterior tibial muscle (especially if the child has a very flat foot).

Traction of the navicular tuberosity from tibialis posterior tendon can cause:

- tendinopathy,
- posterior tibial tendon dysfunction
- fractures.

The morphology of the navicular is variable. The wider or *cornate* navicular may alter the stability of the tarsus if the agonist–antagonist relationship between tibialis posterior and the peroneal group is disrupted (common in the pronated foot or with ankle equinus). A prominent navicular may be indicative of an accessory navicular or *os tibiale externum* which is found in 10% of the population (Drennan 1992; Fig. 13.7).

Fifth metatarsal

Fractures of note are:

- Jones (metaphyseal region of styloid process, prone to non-union and often requires internal fixation)
- neck
- base (avulsion via peroneus brevis attachment)
- shaft (diaphyseal, the dancer's fracture).

Iselin's disease

This is a traction apophysitis of the base of the fifth metatarsal at the insertion point of peroneus brevis and a lateral slip of the plantar fascia. It is due to excessive tension or repeated blows. Found in ages 10–14 years, it sometimes coexists with Sever's disease. It is necessary to differentiate from a fracture or the accessory bone of this location, the

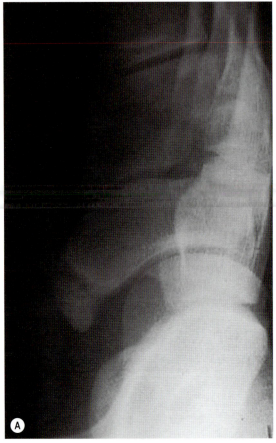

Figure 13.7 Navicular conditions. (A) Os tibiale externum in a young adult.

os vesalianum, which is found in less than 1% of the population (Fig. 13.8).

Clinically, there is tenderness of the fifth metatarsal styloid process. This may be increased by testing peroneus brevis against resistance. Like Sever's disease, Iselin's is largely a clinical diagnosis, but X-rays clarify this apophysis (from a flake fracture or the os vesalianum).

Management includes the RICER approach and stretching the peroneal muscles is helpful, especially in the pronated foot where this group

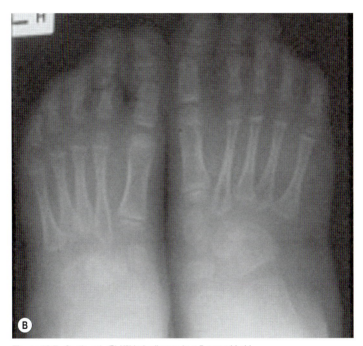

Figure 13.7 *Continued.* (B) Köhler's disease in a 5-year-old girl.

is often tight. Shoes need to be selected so that the basic footwear construction (or template *last*) matches the foot type. A curved last shoe can aggravate the fifth metatarsal base in a rectus (straight) foot type. Basic foot biomechanics may need to be addressed in some cases: e.g. a supinated foot type may overload the fifth metatarsal base; a pronated foot type may have tight peroneals which are unopposed by a functionally disadvantaged tibialis posterior.

Buschke's disease

This is a very rare entity, an osteochondrosis of a cuneiform. Buschke's *disease* can affect any of the cuneiforms. It affects children aged 4–6 years and boys are predisposed. Presentation includes midfoot pain, sometimes only with increased activity levels. Shape of cuneiform is abnormal for age on X-ray (Fig. 13.9).

Treatment depends upon the symptoms and activity level of the child. A below-knee walking cast is usually applied for 4–6 weeks.

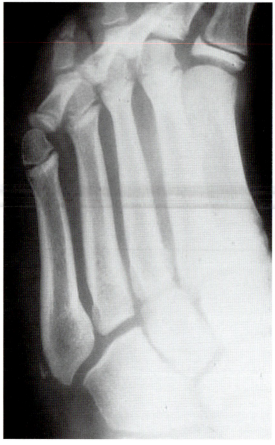

Figure 13.8 Iselin's disorder or osteochondrosis of the fifth metatarsal apophysis. The os vesalianum is present in approximately 1% of the population and is less likely to be associated with symptoms in this area.

Forefoot

Freiberg's infraction

This is an articular subchondral osteochondrosis of a metatarsal head. Freiberg's usually occurs after 12 years of age and usually affects the second, third or fourth metatarsal heads (Fig. 13.10). Girls are more com-

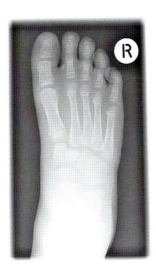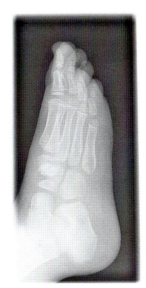

Figure 13.9 Buschke's disease. Osteochondrosis of the intermediate cuneiform in a 7-year-old boy. Note the sclerosis and 'shrinkage' from the margins.

monly affected than boys and the age range is approximately 12–15 years.

Radiology reveals a collapse of the articular surface of the affected metatarsal head (most commonly the longer second metatarsal, especially in a Morton's foot type).

Clinically, there is dorsal tenderness of the second metatarsal head (68% of cases), of the third metatarsal head (27% of cases), or unusually the fourth metatarsal head (5% of cases) (Bloomfield et al 1992). The range of the affected joint is reduced and painful to elicit.

Management of Freiberg's *disease* includes:

- RICER – to settle the acute phase
- stretching – tight triceps surae unload the heel and load the forefoot
- shoes – forefoot cushioning, especially for high-impact sports
- biomechanics – a Morton's foot type (short first ray) may predispose the second metatarsal head.

The main differential diagnosis to include is a stress fracture. These are particularly common in ballet dancers and aerobic participants. Later

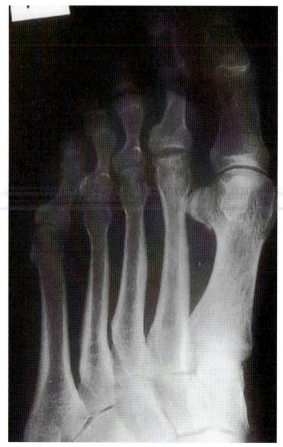

Figure 13.10 Freiberg's infraction. Osteochondrosis of the second metatarsal head with noticeable flattening and osteophytic margins. This 64-year-old male recalled having a very sore forefoot as a teenager and having to rest from playing basketball for a season.

implications include a propensity towards osteoarthritis of the affected joint.

Hallux valgus

This is a common orthopaedic foot problem for which there is often a strong family history.

The best management of juvenile hallux valgus is uncertain. Foot orthoses have been found not to slow progression of the deformity (Kilmartin & Wallace 1992). There are over 100 different surgical techniques described for hallux valgus and a 10% recurrence rate associated with surgical correction (Deenik et al 2008).

Conservative management is clinically based and includes:

- footwear advice
- mobilizing the first metatarsophalangeal joint
- splinting (Fig. 13.11).

In my experience, these measures can alleviate mild symptoms, as can the judicious use of foot orthoses, which address abnormal biomechanics. It is important to be realistic about treatment options with young people and not to evade the likelihood of progression of the deformity.

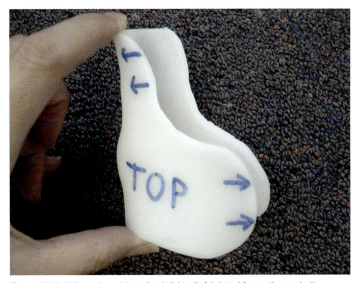

Figure 13.11 Hallux valgus night splint. Individually fabricated from a thermoplastic sheeting this splint is attached across the metatarsal heads and around the hallux with 1–2 cm elastic. It is worn at night-time and clinical experience has found it helpful in reducing hallux abduction, especially if the child also mobilizes the joint and exercises abductor hallucis.

Family history, connective tissue properties, weight and activity levels seem to be/may be relevant factors. Symptomatic cases often require surgery and cosmesis can be a very distressing issue for girls.

References

Accadbled F, Laville J-M, Harper L 2003 One-step treatment for evolved Blount's disease. Journal of Pediatric Orthopedics 23(6):747–752

Alfredson H, Cook J 2007 A treatment algorithm for managing Achilles tendinopathy: a new treatment option. British Journal of Sports Medicine 41(4):211–216

Aparaicio G, Abril JC, Alvarez L 1997 Radiologic study of patellar height in Osgood–Schlatter disease. Journal of Pediatric Orthopedics 17:63–66

Bloomfield J, Fricker PA, Fitch KD 1992 Textbook of science and medicine in sport. Blackwell Scientific Publications, Melbourne

Brukner P, Khan K 1993 Clinical sports medicine. McGraw-Hill, Sydney

Crawford DC, Safran MR 2006 Osteochondritis dissecans of the knee. Journal of the American Academy of Orthopaedic Surgeons 14(2):90–100

Deenik AR, de Visser E, Louwerens J-WK 2008 Hallux valgus angle as main predictor for correction of hallux valgus. BMC Musculoskeletal Disorders 9:70–75

Demirag BA, Ozturk CA, Yazici ZB et al 2004 The pathophysiology of Osgood–Schlatter disease: a magnetic resonance investigation. Journal of Pediatric Orthopedics 13(6):379

Drennan JC 1992 The child's foot and ankle. Raven Press, New York

Dyment PG 1991 The sports physical. Adolescent Medicine 2(1):1–12

Eckerwall G, Lohmander LS, Windstrand H 1997 Increased levels of proteoglycan fragments and stromelysin in hip joint fluid in Legg–Calvé–Perthes disease. Journal of Pediatric Orthopedics 17(2):266–269

Evans AM 2001a Heel pain is not always plantar fasciitis or a 'spur' – consider the spectrum. Sport Health 19(4):17–19

Evans AM 2001b Osteochondroses of the foot. Sport Health 19(3):20–22

Evans AM, Scutter S, Iasiello H 2003 Sonographic investigation of the paediatric navicular – an exploratory study in four year old children. Journal of Diagnostic Medical Sonography 19(4):217–221

Frank JB, Jarit GJ, Bravman JT 2007 Lower extremity injuries in the skeletally immature athlete. Journal of the American Academy of Orthopaedic Surgeons 15(6):356–366

Galli M, Crivellini M, Santambrogio GC et al 2001 Short-term effects of 'botulinum toxin A' as treatment for children with cerebral palsy: kinematic and kinetic aspects at the ankle joint. Functional Neurology 16(4):317–323

Gigante A, Bevilacqua C, Bonetti MG et al 2003 Increased external tibial torsion in Osgood–Schlatter disease. Acta Orthopaedica Scandinavica 74(4):431–436

Gould JA 1990 Orthopaedic and sports physical therapy, 2nd edn. Mosby, St Louis

Handoll HHG, Rowe BH, Quinn KM et al 2001 Interventions for preventing ankle ligament injuries. Cochrane Database of Systematic Reviews 2001:(3)

Kilmartin TE, Wallace WA 1992 The significance of pes planus in juvenile hallux valgus. Foot and Ankle 13(2):53–56

Menz HB, Munteanu SE 2005 Radiographic validation of the Manchester scale for the classification of hallux valgus deformity. Rheumatology 44:1061–1066

Myers MT, Thompson GH 1997 Imaging the child with a limp. Pediatric Clinics of North America 44(3):637–658

Ogden JA, Ganey TM, Hill JD et al 2004 Sever's injury: a stress fracture of the immature calcaneal metaphysis. Journal of Pediatric Orthopedics 24(5):488–492

Ross MD, Villard D 2003 Disability levels of college-aged men with a history of Osgood–Schlatter disease. Journal of Strength Conditioning Research 17(4):659–663

Saraph V, Zwick EB, Ernst B et al 2001 Conservative management of dynamic equinus in diplegic children treated by gait improvement surgery. Journal of Pediatric Orthopedics B 10(4):287–292

Sarrafian SK 1993 Anatomy of the foot and ankle, 2nd edn. JB Lippincott, Philadelphia

Scuderi GR, McCann PD 2005 Sports medicine: a comprehensive approach, 2nd edn. Elsevier Mosby, Philadelphia

Seeman E 1996 Pathogenesis of osteoporosis in the first 20 years of life: a review. Australian Specialist 2(1):9–11

Sports Medicine Australia 2008 Safety guidelines for children in sport and recreation, 2nd edn. ACT Mitchell, Sports Medicine Australia

Tardieu C, Lespargot A, Tabary C et al 1988 For how long must the soleus muscle be stretched each day to prevent contracture? Developmental Medicine and Child Neurology 30(1):3–10

Further reading

American Academy of Pediatrics: www.aap.org

Smartplay – injury prevention fact sheets/ guidelines/ injury prevention research: www.smartplay.com.au

Sports Medicine Australia: www.sma.org.au

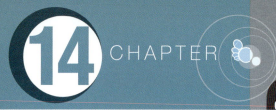

14 CHAPTER

Footwear

Why we wear shoes

Since ancient times, people have protected their feet against the elements and rough terrain. Animal skins were used to cover the feet, lashed securely above the ankle in a crude, but effective, moccasin style. Other than for protection when walking, footwear was not used and the feet of our nomadic ancestors grew strong from coping with uneven surfaces, climbing trees, swimming in streams and scaling rock faces.

Today, footwear is as much about aesthetic appearance as basic protection (Cowell 1977, Staheli 1994). Fashion dictates the footwear people choose and it is remarkable to see the level of discomfort people will endure in order to achieve the successfully marketed 'look'. While women are the main group to suffer as footwear fashion victims (and it can be hard to find comfortable female fashion footwear that looks good), children are not immune either. Rampant consumerism and large-scale manu-facturing of footwear has seen a huge change in the supply and style of footwear in the last 50 years (ask your older patients what type and how many pairs of shoes they had as an 8-year-old and compare that with many chil-dren now). Status is another aspect of foot-wear selection and of course the foot fetishists are not to be overlooked (Stewart 1972).

Attitudes have changed. While many parents are still diligent about their children's shoes, many are unaware and blasé, not having experienced post-war rationing and having to wear shoes that were too small because they could not afford or access new ones. Children are now far more actively involved in choosing their wardrobes and daily attire, including shoes. So, of course, the pretty sparkling fairy slip-ons and the Superhero Loafers with flashing lights are going to appeal more than the black/brown laced school shoes. Worn down, busy parents (who may not have even a basic knowledge of foot growth) will often understandably relent to the mass marketing pressure dispensed through their offspring.

Key *Concepts*

> There is a relative dearth of education about and research into children's footwear, when we consider the scale of the issue.

There are many long-held opinions, e.g. that trainers/runners are not good for children's feet, that are too general and not well founded. The selection of children's footwear for general purpose and the fit of that shoe are probably more important than the periodic use of party shoes. It is really a matter of *horses for courses*.

What is known about the effects of shoes on children's feet

Children's footwear which incorporates arch support has been demonstrated to hasten the development of the medial foot arch if worn between ages 1 and 3 years (Gould et al 1989). The same study showed that arch development was the same by age 5 years, independent of footwear type.

Key *Concepts*

> A randomized controlled trial showed no difference in the arch profile of flexible flat foot with the use of corrective shoes or foot orthoses in children aged 1–6 years (Cohen & Cowell 1989, Wenger et al 1989).

This finding has also been supported (with less scientific rigour) by other investigators (Mereday et al 1972, Penneau et al 1982).

Large studies in India have found correlation between the use of footwear and the incidence of flat feet in children (Gould et al 1989, Rao & Joseph 1992, Sachithanandam & Joseph 1995). It is clearly a leap to assume that these results transpose across to cultures where footwear and hard surfaces now predominate.

The effects of shoes on children's gait

The effects of putting shoes on children has been examined in different age groups and settings. An Australian study examined the effects of sneakers and Clarks first walker shoes versus bare feet on the gait of 31 children (aged 13–32 months, mean 19 months; Wilkinson 1997). The main findings were:

- Initial effects were greater for shoes than for sneakers:
  - increased ankle dorsiflexion
  - increased base of gait
  - reduced angle of gait.
- Shoes and sneakers had different effects:
  - sneakers produced ankle plantarflexion during swing phase.
- Children adapted to the effects of new footwear in less than 1 month:
  - the sole of shoes became more flexible with use
  - gait matured and changed aside from footwear use.

The effects of footwear on normal children in a gait laboratory found no kinetic or kinematic differences but found that wearing shoes increased stride length. As a result, it has been suggested that barefoot gait may be sufficient for most clinical studies (Oeffinger et al 1999).

A Congolese study assessed footprint data in 1851 children (aged 3–12 years). The children were from both rural and urban environments and had differing exposure to footwear, from never worn to always worn. It was concluded that footwear had very little influence on foot morphology (age and gender were the predictive factors) (Echarri & Forriol 2003, Pfeiffer et al 2006).

A recent study from Germany has looked at the effects of conventional versus more flexible shoes in the gait patterns of 8-year-old children. There were significant changes in the position and motion of the medial foot arch when conventional footwear was used. Motion was generally restricted in comparison to barefoot gait. The study concluded that more flexible footwear allowed foot motion that was more like that occurring when barefoot as opposed to when wearing more 'supportive' shoes (Wolf et al 2008).

Foot growth and shoe size

Key Concepts

Foot growth in children aged 1–5 years has been studied prospectively and found to correlate inversely with age, i.e. the feet of younger children grow faster than the feet of older children (Gould et al 1990).

Clearly this has implications for shoe size. Toddlers may need to change shoe size every 2 months, although this is variable. Little feet are very pliable, so it is easy to keep them in shoes that are too small, as the toes buckle with little force to fit into a cramped space.

Measuring children's feet has long been regarded as an important practice. Ensuring that children have shoes that fit well and, by inference, will not damage the feet and yet allow for growth is particularly important. The length, width and depth of each foot needs to be assessed and then shoes selected to match these parameters and also those of style, price, preference and purpose. Shoe-fitting for children is not easy and an experienced fitter of children's shoes is both skilled and necessarily patient. Personally, as a clinician, I have found this an invaluable liaison.

Measuring the size of the foot

As part of the undergraduate podiatry programme in Adelaide, Australia, final year students completed a shoe-fitting course courtesy of Clarks Australia (also provided by Clarks in the UK). One of the components of this course included the practical use of foot measure devices, commonly used in retail stores (Fig. 14.1).

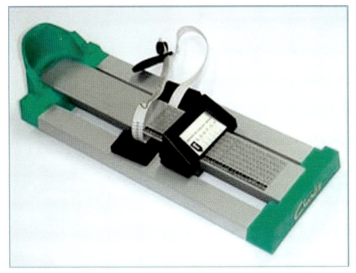

Figure 14.1 The foot measure used in the reliability study and used commercially in shoe retail outlets.

The reliability of this foot size measuring technique was subsequently evaluated as a clinical research pilot study using a same subject repeated measures study design. The sample was one of convenience ($n = 14$), with podiatry students ($n = 6$, ages 20–25 years) and paediatric clinic patients ($n = 8$, ages 5–12 years). The examiners were two final year podiatry students and two podiatry teaching staff. All had attended the same shoe-fitting course. Results are found in Table 14.1 (Evans & Carty 2007).

This pilot study indicated that all examiners were very reliable at measuring foot length. The reliability of foot width (girth) measures was less. Hence the combined foot length and width measures were also less reliable. These trends were largely consistent both within and between examiners, and regardless of professional experience. Implications include the accuracy of width versus length shoe fittings, foot growth studies, training of retail shoe-fitting staff.

In a large study of 2829 Chinese children, feet were found to grow linearly from age 3 to age 12 in girls and from age 3 to age 15 in boys. Growth was more than linear in both genders when children were aged less than 2 years and later plateaued, after linear growth cessation. Children's feet increased in both length and width when standing, which is clearly relevant for the measuring and fitting of feet in shoes. An

Table 14.1 Reliability of foot size measures

The examiners were two students and two clinical staff, all of whom were trained to measure foot size at the same workshop. As can be seen, the measure of length was highly reliable across all examiners, but width (girth) measures were much less reliable

Foot size measure	Examiner 1 (student)	Examiner 2 (student)	Examiner 3 (staff)	Examiner 4 (staff)
Intra-rater ICC (1,1)	Left right	Left right	Left right	Left right
Foot length	0.99 0.99	0.99 0.99	0.99 0.05*	0.99 0.99
Foot width	0.81 0.90	0.47 0.82	0.75 0.47	0.81 0.74
Foot length and width	0.41 0.41	0.30 0.33	0.31 0.29^	0.62 0.58
Inter-rater ICC (1,1)				
Foot length	Left = 0.99		Right = 0.99**	
Foot width	Left = 0.52		Right = 0.61	
Foot length and width	Left = 0.42		Right = 0.43**	

*Examiner 3 (staff) missed two subjects' right foot length measures.
**Examiner 3's right foot length measures excluded.

increase of between 2.1 and 4.4 mm was noted when the feet were weight-bearing.

Shoes for new walkers, older children

Considering the possible permutations when fitting children's shoes is somewhat akin to *Goldilocks*' experience of sampling the three bears porridge – there are shoes that are:

- too short – cause toes to curl or hurt
- too narrow – rub and hurt
- too wide – slip, rub and hurt
- too long – increase tripping
- just right – protect a child's foot, are comfortable to wear, but will soon be too small!

The quest for well-fitting footwear for children is ongoing throughout childhood, if there is to be a happy ending (Fig. 14.2).

The best-available criteria for selecting a shoe for a new walking child are:

- Fitted with the child standing.
- Allow for growth of half a size for largest foot.
- Flexible sole at forefoot.
- Securing mechanism, e.g. laces, strap/buckle, Velcro straps.

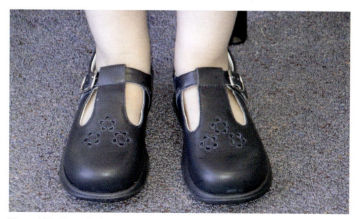

Figure 14.2 Shoe selection factors for children's first shoes.

A survey of the factors which influence parents when choosing footwear for their children revealed that the following criteria are considered:

- comfort
- quality
- climatic season
- health professional advice.

Interestingly, cost of footwear was found to be of only moderate or no interest (Wilkinson 1997).

Key *Concepts*

Considering the increase in self-service shoe outlets for children's shoes, providing educational material and guidelines for parents could be very beneficial.

Specific footwear issues

Heelys

A relatively recent innovation and potentially great fun, the use of Heelys may be made safer with some greater use of protective gear and better supervision during the learning phase. Most injuries sustained from using Heelys are upper limb fractures in novice gliders (Vioreanu et al 2007).

New football boots

There have been recent reports of toxic shock from blistering over the Achilles tendon due to *Staphylococcus aureus* infection in children wearing new football boots (Taylor et al 2006).

Key *Concepts*

Toxic shock is unusual in children and a serious consequence of blistering from footwear. Any abrasions resulting from the use of new football/rugby boots should therefore be taken seriously.

Equestrian foot injuries

Midfoot injuries are more common in children undertaking equestrian activity. Lisfranc dislocations, complex midfoot fractures and fractures of the cuboid, talus, metatarsals, tibial malleolus and joint displacements have all been reported. Safety stirrups, stronger boots and close supervision may reduce some of these potentially disabling injuries (Ceroni et al 2007).

Special cases

Cerebral palsy

The use of hinged ankle foot orthoses (AFOs) has been found to benefit children with cerebral palsy (diplegia) by requiring reduced oxygen and pulmonary ventilatory costs by approximately 10% (Maltais et al 2001; Fig. 14.3).

Key *Concepts*

> Hinged AFOs have also been shown to facilitate increased ankle power and better ankle dorsiflexion in comparison with solid AFOs (Radtka et al 2006).

The use of wedged shoes with AFOs may assist children with cerebral palsy who crouch (Wesdock & Edge 2003).

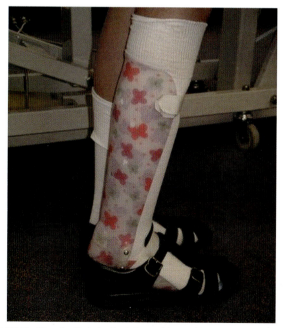

Figure 14.3 The hinged ankle foot orthosis for an 11-year-old girl with right-side hemiplegia. Comfort, stability and energy efficiency are prime considerations for these children.

Figure 14.4 shows a 21-month-old child with hemiplegia. Boots can help to stabilize, but are often insufficient to stabilize against altered muscle tone. A supplementary AFO was required to establish better weight transfer to the affected side.

Developmental delay (George & Elchert 2007)

Stabilizing foot splints are largely used for children with gait and function difficulties according to clinical experience (see Ch. 15). A case study of

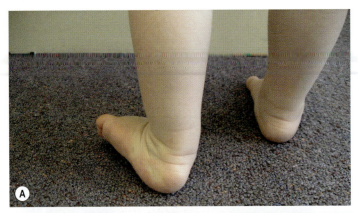

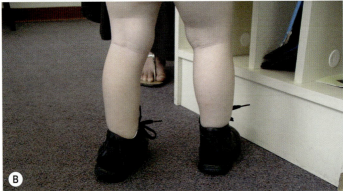

Figure 14.4 (A) Child with left-side hemiplegia, aged 21 months, pulling to stand, not walking unaided.
(B) Insufficient support from boots alone. This child required a supramalleolar ankle foot orthosis for her left foot, in order to establish a stable independent stance and gait.

a 19-month-old child with hypotonia and developmental delay, due to hydrocephalus and congenital absence of the corpus callosum, assessed the use of stabilizing foot splints (SFSs). Motor performance (e.g. rise-to-stand, cruising, stepping) were assessed using a motor skills scale when the child was barefoot, wearing shoes, wearing shoes and SFSs. These observations were made across a 3-week time span and found that the child's performance was most improved when wearing the shoes and SFSs. A larger-scale study of SFSs as an intervention is warranted (George & Elchert 2007).

Much of the use of footwear and foot orthoses in children with special needs is based upon clinical impression. While this is valuable, practical and rich data, the aspects of scientific studies which reduce the likelihood of chance findings are lacking (such as adequate sample size, randomization, control group comparison). The use of single case experimental design (SCED) and the patient generated index (PGI) are practical and feasible in these situations and greatly improve the strength of findings (Ch. 6). Clinicians are encouraged to adopt these methods into their practice. This author has found both SCED and PGI to be easily incorporated into regular practice and invaluable for better discerning outcomes (Evans 2003).

Psychological issues and footwear

The issue of children's foot problems and footwear has been largely approached from a physical functioning perspective. While this is understandable, it also reflects the emphasis and the compartmentalizing of people's health care as opposed to an all-encompassing holistic model.

Quality of life (QoL) measures are now recognized as pivotal in the recognition and management of health (Carr & Higginson 2001). The World Health Organization (WHO) emphasizes QoL measures in epidemiological surveys and large-scale intervention projects (WHO 2007). Children's pain experiences are well-researched fields and the psychological effects of pain are validated (McGrath et al 2000).

Key *Concepts*

Modified shoe use during childhood has been correlated with lower self-esteem in later life. In addition, adults who wore special shoes as children recalled: decreased self-image, teasing about their shoes, limitation of activities and a generally negative experience (Driano et al 1998).

Acknowledging that many children are affected by foot and ankle problems, a questionnaire to assess the wider health and social costs has been developed (Morris et al 2007). Using focus groups for children with a variety of foot problems across age groups elicited the following main findings:

- activity was more difficult
- physical pain
- reduced participation (in life activities)
- self-consciousness.

The complexity of these issues increased with age and the most common focus for self-consciousness was footwear. Children and parents described strategies to hide the wearing of foot orthoses. Children over 8 years of age were much more self-conscious of their footwear

References

Carr AJ, Higginson IJ 2001 Are quality of life measures patient centred? BMJ 322(7298):1357–1360

Ceroni D, De Rosa V, De Coulon G et al 2007 The importance of proper shoe gear and safety stirrups in the prevention of equestrian foot injuries. Journal of Foot and Ankle Surgery 46(1):32–39

Cohen J, Cowell HR 1989 Corrective shoes [editorial]. Journal of Bone and Joint Surgery – American Volume 71(6):799

Cowell HR 1977 Shoes and shoe corrections. Pediatric Clinics of North America 24(4):791–797

Driano AN, Staheli L, Staheli LT 1998 Psychological development and corrective shoewear use in childhood. Journal of Pediatric Orthopedics 18(3):346–349

Echarri JJ, Forriol F 2003 The development in footprint morphology in 1851 Congolese children from urban and rural areas, and the relationship between this and wearing shoes. Journal of Pediatric Orthopedics 12(2):141–146

Evans AM 2003 Relationship gretween 'growing pains' and foot posture in children: single-case experimental designs in clinical practice. Journal of the American Podiatric Medical Association 93(2):111

Evans AM, Carty MM 2007 Reliability of measuring children's foot size. Book of Abstracts. 22nd Australasian Podiatry Conference. [Abstract]

George DA, Elchert L 2007 The influence of foot orthoses on the function of a child with developmental delay. Pediatric Physical Therapy 19(4):332–336

Gould N, Moreland M, Alvarez R et al 1989 Development of the child's arch. Foot and Ankle 9(5):241–245

Gould N, Moreland M, Trevino S et al 1990 Foot growth in children aged one to five years. Foot and Ankle 10(4):211–213

McGrath PA, Speechley KN, Seifert CE et al 2000 A survey of children's acute, recurrent, and chronic pain: validation of the pain experience interview. Pain 87(1):59–73

Maltais D, Bar-Or O, Galea V et al 2001 Use of orthoses lowers the O(2) cost of walking in children with spastic cerebral palsy. Medicine and Science in Sports and Exercise 33(2):320–325

Mereday C, Dolan CM, Lusskin R 1972 Evaluation of the University of California Biomechanics Laboratory shoe insert in 'flexible' pes planus. Clinical Orthopaedics and Related Research 82:45–58

Morris C, Liabo K, Wright P et al 2007 Development of the Oxford ankle foot questionnaire: finding out how children are affected by foot and ankle problems. Child Care and Health Development 33(5):559–568

Oeffinger D, Braunch B, Cranfill S et al 1999 Comparison of gait with and without shoes in children. Gait Posture 9(2):95–100

Penneau K, Lutter LD, Winter RB 1982 Pes planus radiographic changes with foot orthoses and shoes. Foot and Ankle 2:299–303

Pfeiffer M, Kotz R, Ledl T et al 2006 Prevalence of flat foot in preschool-aged children. Pediatrics 118(2):634–639

Radtka SA, Oliveira GB, Lindstrom KE et al 2006 The kinematic and kinetic effects of solid, hinged, and no ankle-foot orthoses on stair locomotion in healthy adults. Gait Posture 24(2):211–218

Rao UB, Joseph B 1992 The influence of footwear on the prevalence of flat foot: a survey of 2300 children [see comments]. Journal of Bone and Joint Surgery – British Volume 74(4):525–527

Sachithanandam V, Joseph B 1995 The influence of footwear on the prevalence of flat foot: a survey of 1846 skeletally mature persons. Journal of Bone and Joint Surgery – British Volume 77(2):254–257

Staheli LT 1994 Footwear for children. [Review] [50 refs]. Instructional Course Lectures 43:193–197

Stewart SF 1972 Footgear – its history and abuses. Clinical Orthopedics and Related Research 88:119–130

Taylor CM, Riordan FAI, Graham C 2006 New football boots and toxic shock syndrome. BMJ (332):1376–1378

Vioreanu M, Sheehan E, Glynn A et al 2007 Heelys and street gliders injuries: a new type of pediatric injury. Pediatrics 119(6):e1294–e1298

Wenger DR, Mauldin D, Speck G et al 1989 Corrective shoes and inserts as treatment for flexible flatfoot in infants and children [see comments]. Journal of Bone and Joint Surgery – American Volume 71(6):800–810

Wesdock KA, Edge AM 2003 Effects of wedged shoes and ankle-foot orthoses on standing balance and knee extension in children with cerebral palsy who crouch. Pediatric Physical Therapy 15(4):221–231

Wilkinson MJ 1997 The effects of footwear on selected parameters of gait in early independent walking. La Trobe University, Bundoora, Victoria, Australia

Wolf S, Simon J, Patikas D et al 2008 Foot motion in children shoes: a comparison of barefoot walking with shod walking in conventional and flexible shoes. Gait Posture 27(1):51–59

World Health Organization. The world health report – 2007: a safer future. World Health Organization, Geneva

Orthoses

Introduction

This is largely an experienced-based clinical chapter. In particular, Table 15.1 outlines my professional opinion and experience with various orthoses for a range of clinical presentations.

Footwear selection is often fundamental and intrinsic to the use of foot orthoses and in-shoe wedging and also for the use of torsional splints (Ch. 14).

Footwear and attached splints are also an integral part of the management of metatarsus adductus (Ch. 9) and talipes equinovarus (Ch. 8).

Key Concepts

The efficacy and benefit of foot orthoses for adults is not in doubt (Landorf & Keenan 2000). Much less is known, however, about the value of foot orthoses for children, in whom there is well-founded concern about unnecessary and expensive use of foot orthoses (Pfeiffer et al 2006; Rome et al 2006; Staheli 1987, 1999; Wenger et al 1989; Whitford & Esterman 2007).

Classification of children's flat foot types assists the clinical decision-making process regarding development, monitoring and treatment need or options. Using the paediatric flat foot proforma (p-FFP; Evans 2007) may clarify this

Table 15.1 Summary of various orthotic devices used in the author's clinical practice

	Indication	Child's age	Benefits	Pitfalls
Torsional splints				
Denis Browne splint	1. Lower leg torsion/position 2. Post casting: TEV/MTA	0–5 0–3 (MTA) 0–10 (TEV)	Strong, durable	Heavy
Ganley splint	1. Lower leg torsion/ position 2. Post casting: TEV/MTA	0–3 (MTA) 0–4 (TEV)	Provides positioning of forefoot to rear foot	Time-consuming to fit; unattractive metallic bars/plates
Counter rotation splint	1. Lower leg torsion/position 2. Post casting: TEV/MTA	0–4 0–4	Hinged bar allows motion, well tolerated	No longer available; easily broken; expensive but best accepted
Unibar	1. Lower leg torsion/position 2. Post casting: TEV/MTA	0–4 0–4	360° positioning of foot to bar; lightweight	Not easily available
Fillauer bar	1. Lower leg torsion/position 2. Post casting: TEV/MTA	0–5 0–3 (MTA) 0–10 (TEV)	Clips onto existing footwear	Heavy; clamps often tear sheets
Wheaton brace	1. MTA 2. TEV 3. Calcaneovalgus 4. Intoe, out-toe	0–2	Does not attach the feet in the manner of bars Can address single foot problems	Not always a sufficiently specific fit; can be hot to wear
Other splints and devices				
NSS	Equinus	4–15	Maintains ankle position at rest, yet removable Can adjust ankle position/time	Can be hot to wear. Variable comfort reported

		Need to be old enough to manage necessary gait adaptation		
Cast walker	# e.g. 5th met Ankle inv injury Sever's		Maintains activity and bone stress, yet immobilizes rear foot regions	Must even up limb length with contralateral shoe
Customized foot wedging, orthoses and splints				
Triplane wedges	Non-developmental flat feet, hypotonia, hypermobility	1–5	Cheap, simple, effective	Glued into one pair of shoes
Gait plates	Intoe with tripping, falling	3–10	Cheap simple, often effective	Need a flexible sole shoe
Thermoplastics, e.g. Aquaplast	Hypermobile flat foot Mild hemiplegia Mild ankle equinus Hallux valgus	1–6	Individualized, easy application for hypermobile feet and mild neuromotor tone cases	Takes some practice to perfect fabrication; not durable
Customized foot orthoses (from foot cast/scan)	Not generally required in children under 10 years		Addresses asymmetry e.g. hemiplegia, size, deformity, trauma. Can use very durable materials	Expensive
Prefabricated foot wedging, orthoses				
Valgus wedges	Variation on triplane wedges	1–5	Cheap, simple, effective	Need to be well positioned to avoid rubbing
Heel cups	Rear foot instability	1–3	Rear foot instability (often hypermobile new or late walkers) when footwear support is beneficial but insufficient	Quickly outgrown (6/12). Require well-secured shoes as movement irritates. Tendency for slippage

Continued

Table 15.1 Summary of various orthotic devices used in the author's clinical practice – cont'd

	Indication	Child's age	Benefits	Pitfalls
Prefabricated foot wedging, orthoses				
Heel raises	Sever's and equinus – sport Sx – hemiplegia	8–14	Provide quick reduction of calcaneal apophysis traction and resulting symptoms of Sever's cases	Should only be used to alleviate initial symptoms and for sport. Full-time use contributes to equinus
Prefabricated foot orthoses ¾ (a) rearfoot	Rear foot compensations (NWB rear foot to forefoot congruent)	5–15 +	Quick, cheap, effective. Can be adapted with extrinsic posting	Sand in shoes reduces durability – advise parents to empty shoes. Leave forefoot space if sock liner is removed (easily filled)
Prefabricated foot orthoses F/L (b) midfoot	Forefoot compensations (NWB rearfoot to leg basically congruent)	5–15 +	Quick, cheap, effective. Can be adapted with extrinsic posting. Do not move in shoes which is 'anti-blistering' for sports	Do not always transfer well between different shoe styles due to specific full-length trim. Less durable than ¾ length style (not a big issue when considering foot growth)

AJ = ankle jerk
F/L = full length
HAV = hallux valgus
met = metatarsal
MTA = metatarsus adductus.
NWB = non-weight-bearing.
SX = symptom
TEV = talipes equinovarus.

sometimes murky and poorly rationalized process for clinicians and parents (see Ch. 6). While less common, excessive supination may also require foot orthoses.

Splints, boots and in-shoe orthoses

Splints (and bars)

By definition, splints are used to hold a structural position with the rationale of moulding or training these structural tissues into the held position.

The saying 'just as the twig is bent, so is the tree inclined' (attributed to Alexander Pope) was long held to be true by clinicians and underpinned the prescription of physical limb and foot splinting for decades (Evans 2007; Ganley 1984, 1987; Kite 1967). The ability of tissues to respond (stress, strain, form and deform) is not in question here; it is a basic physical property. However, the use of externally applied and worn splints to intrinsically alter foot and leg morphology is well disputed and hence the current decline of the use of most orthopaedic splints. An exception to this is the use of the Ilizarov bone pin external fixation devices which apply forces direct to osseous tissues and are used for fractures, bony torsions, bone length deficits (applied with adjusted tractioning) (Herzenberg et al 1994).

Alongside the questioning of splint efficacy, there has also emerged better knowledge and understanding of the normal developmental trends which exist in the paediatric population: for example, in the past orthopaedic clinics have been quite keen to treat children who presented with an intoeing gait and Denis Browne bars were frequently dispensed to correct the presumed deformity of (medial/internal) tibial torsion. We now question this approach on four main grounds:

1. Some 30% of children under 4 years of age intoe (Thackeray & Beeson 1996a, 1996b).
2. Tibial torsion is expected to be neutral at birth (Cusick 1990, Eckhoff & Johnson 1994).
3. Medial genicular (soft tissue) positioning is commonly mistaken for real tibial torsion (Cusick 1990).
4. The normal angle of gait is −8° to +16° (Losel et al 1996).

There are, however, still applications for which splinting is supported. The maintenance splint for babies with clubfoot who are treated with the Ponseti method has been shown to be a critical factor in the success rate of this 'gold standard' technique (Cooper & Dietz 1995; Dobbs et al 2004;

Haft et al 2007; Herzenberg et al 2002; Gupta et al 2008; Morcuende et al 2004, 2005; Ponseti et al 2003, 2006; Thacker et al 2005; see Ch. 8).

Splinting is also widely used in children with muscular hypertonic conditions and cerebral palsy (Allington et al 2002, Galli et al 2001). In these cases the use of splinting is usually aimed at maintaining muscle length, preventing contracture or shortening, and in doing so reducing the intrinsically deforming forces on young bones (Fabry et al 1994, Kumar & MacEwen 1982).

Night stretch splints

The use of rest or stretch splints often worn at night-time can be useful for children with Sever's disease (calcaneal apophysitis), idiopathic toe walking and Achilles tendon strains and shortening (Alvarez et al 2007, Evans 2001, Hemo et al 2006). These splints address sagittal plane positions and range of motion and can be rigid, adjustable or a sock and strap system (see Fig. 11.4).

These splints capitalize on the connective tissue property of 'creep' – its ability to plastically deform under maintained tensile load. The use of a dorsiflexion toe wedge can add further fascial stretch. Some splints have the foot/leg angle adjustable from 20° plantarflexion to 20° dorsiflexion in 10° increments, which allows for increased stretch loading as the range increases.

While the Denis Browne bar has been and remains the mainstay of torsional splints, there have been a number of other popular devices which will be briefly described (Fig. 15.1).

Ganley splint Invented by the late Dr James Ganley DPM (who I was privileged to be hosted and mentored by when studying in Pennsylvania). This is a combination torsion splint with the ability to simultaneously adjust forefoot to rear foot and also foot to leg in all three cardinal body planes. It was designed primarily for the maintenance of metatarsus adductus following corrective serial casting. It can also be used for calcaneovalgus foot deformities and concurrent lower limb rotational problems (Ganley 1984, 1991).

Counter rotation system (CRS) This innovative and almost attractive splint was produced by the Langer Corporation in New York. As the name suggests, this splint addresses lower limb rotations, e.g. intoe. Made of white plastic, the multiple hinged joints made this the most user-friendly splint as, unlike all other anti-torsion splints, the rigid bar was replaced with a mobile framework, allowing more movement and better compliance (Fig. 15.2).

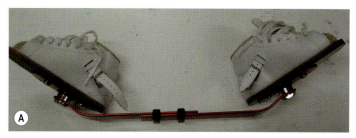

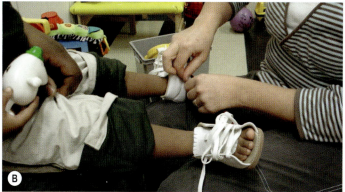

Figure 15.1 (A) Denis Browne bar (bent for clubfoot maintenance).
(B) Fitting a torsion splint with Markell splint boots.

The design was cleverly conceived with detachable foot plates with pivot adjustment for plantarflexion of the first ray. Transverse plane adjustments could be made in 5° increments by adjusting the footplate mountings. There was also provision for unilateral swivel and lock. Tension straps within the frame could further specify the individual rotation range (in eight combinations).

The CRS was expensive and unfortunately prone to breaking, especially at the footplate mounting junction. This was a pity, as in my experience the CRS was second to none in terms of addressing rotational problems. Children tolerated the CRS very well as a night-time splint. Rarely was sleep disruption an issue and many children loved their 'moon boots' (as some called them) and were reluctant to stop wearing them when the treatment was completed. In contrast, the other torsion bars

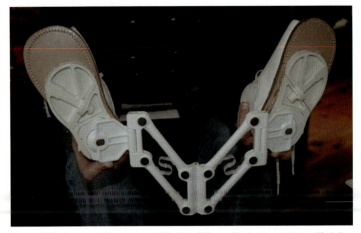

Figure 15.2 Counter rotation system (CRS). This CRS was fitted with straight last Markell splint boots attached to the detachable foot plates. The addition of a triplane or valgus wedge in-shoe reduces rear foot pronation.

are not well tolerated, although much better if started very young as in the case of babies with clubfoot correction using the Ponseti method.

Fillauer bar The Fillauer bar is really an adapted Denis Browne bar which clips onto the child's boots. In theory the child can wear their regular shoes to bed with the splint attached and then it can be removed in the morning. Like the Denis Browne bar, the Fillauer must be bent (approximately 20°) in the frontal plane to protect the feet from forced flattening pronation. The width of the bar should approximate the child's shoulder span to protect the hips from destabilizing as is risked with a narrow bar. Clearly, the bar width must be adjusted for growth.

Unibar This is also a rotational bar but with universal joints attaching the boots to the bar. The unibar also has foot plates which slide off from the bar for attaching and removing. The universal joints allow for three dimensional angulations of each foot. The bar is a lightweight plastic which can be 'snapped' to length with predetermined bar notching.

Wheaton brace This device has numerous cited applications:

- metatarsus adductus
- talipes equinovarus
- calcaneovalgus
- lower limb torsions.

The Wheaton brace does not connect the feet and hence can be used for unilateral and bilateral problems. There are three below-knee designs for metatarsus adductus, talipes equinovarus and calcaneovalgus. A femoral component can be included to address rotation between tibia/fibula and femur.

> ### Key Concepts
>
> The Wheaton brace system allows for many combination deformities to be addressed without the restriction of attaching the feet together (however, knee motion is reduced when the femoral component is used).

The segments are pre-sized which is limiting, but adjustment with heat moulding is possible (see Fig. 9.5). The brace is usually well tolerated by the child except in hot weather when it gets clammy. Some parents find the brace difficult to apply consistently but I have found that opposing markings on the segments usually solve this issue.

Boots

Markell splint boots have long been available for use with rotational splints as outlined below. There are three last styles:

- straight
- inflare
- outflare (see Fig. 15.1).

Usually the straight last boot is worn and if an abductory force is being applied to the feet with a splint, my practice is to insert a triplanar type of in-shoe wedge to negate pronation of the rear foot within the shoe. This is especially important if an outflare style of boot is used, which I have generally only used when abductor hallucis is tight and contributing to atavistic hallux adduction in gait. The straight last boot is my choice in 90% of applications (usually still with triplanar wedging within).

The Markell splint boots can also be used alone, e.g. after splinting has ceased for metatarsus adductus. Many times I have continued to have a child wear their old splint boots at night (detached) for a few months to maintain a non-adducted forefoot position.

Bebax bootees were a great concept but a poor design as the central universal joint slipped or broke regularly. This 3-D boot was great for metatarsus adductus (types 2 and 3) in babies up the age of about 9 months.

Key Concepts

Two simple forget-me-nots

1. Socks

No one ever mentions the basic but important items such as socks and laces. Infants' and children's feet are far easier to get into boots when socks are used. Sock fit needs to keep pace with foot growth, especially in pre-walkers when it is so common to see the toes flexed into bent positions. Parents need to be given general advice about socks, e.g. sizing needs to change according to foot growth (rapid in the first 3 years of life) and socks need to be pulled away from the toes before the feet are put into shoes, as this action always tightens the sock over the toes, flexing or squashing their form (try it yourself when putting on a boot). It is ridiculous for babies and small children to have their foot pushed into socks which are too small (instant confinement) and then to worry about shoe sizing. A more logical approach is:

- measure the feet
- fit the socks (allowing for growth)
- fit the shoes (allowing for growth).

2. Laces

Another common (sense) omission is laces. Boots attached to splints have to be well secured so as not to come off as the child sleeps and moves. Tubular laces are difficult to knot in a way that maintains tension and so tend to come loose and then the shoes come off and the splint use is negated. Flat, ribbon laces tie best and criss-cross threading is my preference for even tension along the boot upper.

In-shoe orthotic supports

Foot orthoses for children can be very useful if prescribed assiduously. It may be timely to review Chapter 6 at this point, in which the development of foot posture and the use of the paediatric flat foot proforma (p-FFP) are discussed.

The first step in using any form of in-shoe orthoses for children is to soundly justify this action. Assessment should be based upon developmental norms, gait parameters and symptoms (if present) and utilize best-tested measures and scales (Evans 2007; Evans & Scutter 2006; Evans et al 2003a, 2003b). Outcome measures need to be decided so that effect can be clinically gauged (Bhatia et al 2004, Carr & Higginson 2001, Evans 2003, Evans et al 2003c, Ruta et al 1994).

A potted history of in-shoe supports

- 1907   Whitman plate
- 1956   Helfet heel seat
- 1967   UCBL (University of California Biomechanics Laboratory) device for flexible flat feet
- 1977   Root orthoses developed (modified versions still prevail)
- 1990   SFS (stabilizing foot splints) for flexible foot deformities
- 2000   An increasing array of useful, inexpensive prefabricated foot orthoses.

The advent of thermoplastics meant that splints could be easily moulded to conform to the foot and leg. These have largely superseded the older-style calipers and boots and provide a functional as opposed to a bracing effect.

Currently there are various approaches to stabilizing a child's foot within a shoe:

a. Triplane wedges

Basically an in-shoe version of the cobbler's 'Thomas heel' which was re-popularized by Valmassy (1996). This is an extremely useful device which when coupled with biomechanical principles and physical laws can effectively and inexpensively improve foot posture and gait. Prefabricated versions exist (e.g. valgus wedges) but it is easy to fashion these from EVA (ethylene vinyl acetate) sheeting (I prefer 10 mm thickness and at least 350 durometer) as Fig. 15.3 illustrates. The positioning of the finished wedge within the shoe is vital for best effect and locating the subtalar joint axis helps to ascertain the site for inducing a supinatory force rather than a pronatory force.

b. Thermoplastics

Aquaplast-T™ is a $\frac{3}{16}$ inch sheet thermoplastic (polypropylene derivative) with the following specifications which make it clinically applicable and useful:

- low-temperature activation – can apply direct to skin (over stockinette)
- rapid set time (child does not have to keep still for long)
- uniform elasticity (allows for conformity around heel and ankle)
- adjustable
- colours (appeal to children, but I find the coloured material has altered properties in comparison with the standard white and that strength and durability are reduced).

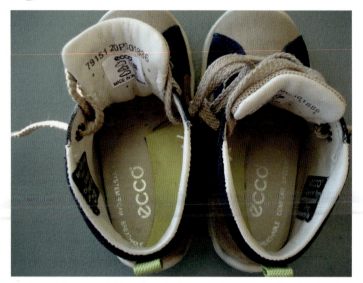

Figure 15.3 The use of simple, inexpensive in-shoe wedges is an effective adjunct for the hypermobile flat foot. Lightweight, yet supportive, flexible footwear is needed to complement the process.

As championed by US physical therapist Beverly Cusick (1990), two styles of Aquaplast splinting which are very useful are described below:

Supramalleolar splints

Also termed DAFO (dynamic ankle foot orthosis), the supramalleolar splints (which as the name suggest include coverage above the ankle malleoli) are typically made from polypropylene pulled very thin over a cast model of the foot and ankle. In effect the DAFO acts more as an exoskeleton and provides some sagittal plane control and greater frontal plane control than regular foot orthoses. The DAFO is often better tolerated than foot orthoses as pressure is spread over a larger skin surface area. The DAFO can provide more stability and control than foot orthoses without using a full AFO (ankle foot orthosis). The DAFO style device can also be made from Aquaplast, in which case it is moulded directly to the foot and ankle, which greatly reduces time and costs.

Indications for a DAFO

- Mild ankle equinus foot deformities, e.g. mild spastic hemiplegia
- Minimal motor dysfunctions, e.g. hypotonia, ligament laxity, i.e. joint hypermobility

- Overt hypotonia
- Suitability for children with spasticity will depend upon:
  - tone
  - static range of motion
  - dynamic range of motion
  - ability to hold foot in a corrected position.

Action (theory) of the supramalleolar splint (DAFO)

- Plantar conformity provides prolonged stretch on short intrinsic foot muscles, which may inhibit tone. This is thought to have a crossover effect on other muscle groups to further and more widely reduce tone.
- Close contact of device with the plantar aspect of the foot provides increased proprioceptive input, which is thought to promote increased postural awareness.
- Better biomechanical alignment may help to promote postural stability.

Stabilizing foot splint (SFS)

An alternative to the UCBL device, the semi weight-bearing fabrication technique of the SFS has the following advantages (Fig. 15.4):

- Calcaneal fat pad is captured in a weighted form.
- Easy visual and tactile positioning.
- 'Friendlier' for the child (who can sit and watch).
- Negates the need for rear foot posting (easier shoe fit).
- Quick to make, fit and dispense.

The principle of the SFS is to prevent deformity and enhance functional gait. It is particularly useful for hypermobile children (regardless of aetiology) and serves as an alternative to triplanar style wedging. Like all orthoses the SFS is very shoe dependent and needs to be well housed and secured for best results and comfort. The Aquaplast SFS is not highly durable (6–12 months) but growth necessitates change within a similar time period.

Prefabricated foot orthoses

The last decade has seen the availability of many useful prefabricated foot orthoses for children. These are quick to instigate and much cheaper than customized orthoses, for which there is no indication in the child presenting with an asymptomatic flat foot (Evans 2007, Harris et al 2004). Many of these 'prefabs' can be adapted to provide more or less support for one or both feet (to a degree). While not as durable as customized orthoses can be, this is seldom an issue as foot growth

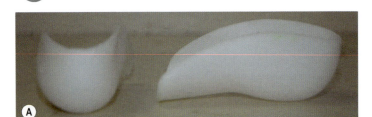

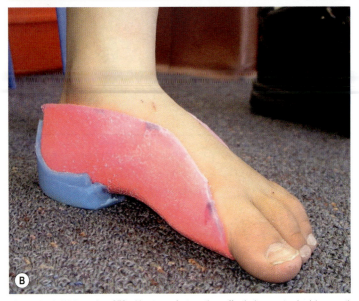

Figure 15.4 (A) Aquaplast SFS without rear foot posting, effectively a customized (non-cast) heel cup. Shoe support is very important to attain gait stability.
(B) Coloured Aquaplast SFS with rear foot posting to increase arch and rear foot stability.

usually necessitates change before material collapse. On average my patients get at least 12–18 months or more from a pair of 'prefabs' at less than 20% the cost of customized foot orthoses. Ethically, we should provide best care for least cost (Fig. 15.5).

Customized foot orthoses

Supported by the scientific evidence, it is this author's opinion and clinical experience that customized foot orthoses are seldom required for children

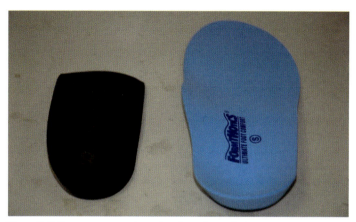

Figure 15.5 There are many good generic orthoses for paediatric use. In general I use styles which address the rear foot (left) and midfoot (right) according to clinical findings.

Table 15.2 An audit of the author's annual orthotic prescribing practice

2007–2008	10 or under	10–16	Over 16	Totals
Foot orthoses	77	139	234	450
a. Generic	65	75	89	229
b. Customized	12	64	145	221

- 51% of all FO were generic, i.e. 229/450
- 66% of customized orthoses were used for patients >16 years, i.e. 145/221
- 61% of generic orthoses were used for children <16 years, i.e. 140/229
- 35% of children <16 years received custom FO, i.e. 76/216
- 15% children <10 years received custom FO, i.e. 12/77

The use of any foot orthoses in young children needs to be reserved for cases who are symptomatic, have delayed/poor gait or wider special needs. Customized foot orthoses are not usually required in children <10 years.

in the first decade of life (Rome et al 2006). The exception to this may be children with rheumatoid arthritis who have been found to be more comfortable and more functional in customized foot orthoses (Powell et al 2005).

Whilst enabling specificity of design, the fabrication of customized foot orthoses is a time-consuming, multi-stage process and thus expensive. Balanced against this, the devices are more durable, accommodate gross asymmetries (e.g. unilateral clubfoot, hemiplegia) and allow for concurrent foot posture and gait angle variations. A recent audit in my practice showed that just 15% of children (less than 10 years) requiring foot orthoses receive customized foot orthoses (an average of one pair per month over 12 months) (Table 15.2). Remember, all of the above-mentioned orthoses are shoe dependent and the combination of shoe/orthotic/foot needs to be appreciated as the child's entire functional unit (see Ch. 14).

References

Allington NJ, Leroy N, Doneux C 2002 Ankle joint range of motion measurements in spastic cerebral palsy children: intraobserver and interobserver reliability and reproducibility of goniometry and visual estimation. Journal of Pediatric Orthopedics B 11(3):236–239

Alvarez C, De Vera M, Beauchamp R et al 2007 Classification of idiopathic toe walking based on gait analysis: development and application of the ITW severity classification. Gait and Posture 26:428–435

Bhatia S, Jenney MEM, Wu E et al 2004 The Minneapolis–Manchester Quality of Life instrument: reliability and validity of the youth form. Journal of Pediatrics 145:39–46

Carr AJ, Higginson IJ 2001 Are quality of life measures patient centred? BMJ 322(7298):1357–1360

Cooper DM, Dietz FR 1995 Treatment of idiopathic clubfoot. Journal of Bone and Joint Surgery – American Volume 77(10):1477–1489

Cusick BD 1990 Progressive casting and splinting for lower extremity deformities in children with neuromotor dysfunction. Therapy Skill Builders, Arizona

Dobbs MB, Rudzki JR, Purcell DB et al 2004 Factors predictive of outcome after use of the Ponseti method for the treatment of idiopathic clubfeet. Journal of Bone and Joint Surgery – American Volume 86(1):22–27

Eckhoff DG, Johnson KK 1994 Three-dimensional computed tomography reconstruction of tibial torsion. Clinical Orthopedics and Related Research (302):42–46

Evans A 2001 Podiatric medical applications of posterior night stretch splinting. Journal of the American Podiatric Medical Association 91(7):356

Evans AM 2003 Relationship between 'growing pains' and foot posture in children: single-case experimental designs in clinical practice. Journal of the American Podiatric Medical Association 93(2):111

Evans AM 2007 The flat footed child – to treat or not to treat, what is the clinician to do? Book of Abstracts, 22nd Australasian Podiatry Conference, pp. 15–16

Evans AM, Scutter S 2006 Sagittal plane range of motion of the pediatric ankle joint: a reliability study. Journal of the American Podiatric Medical Association 96(5):418–422

Evans AM, Copper AW, Scharfbillig RW et al 2003a Reliability of the foot posture index and traditional measures of foot position. Journal of the American Podiatric Medical Association 93(3):203

Evans AM, Scutter SD, Iasiello H 2003b Measuring the paediatric foot: a criterion validity and reliability study of navicular height in 4-year-old children. The Foot 13(2):76–82

Evans A, Scutter S, Lang L 2003c Children's leg pain: development and validation of a parental questionnaire for assessment of prevalence and quality of life (QOL) issues in children aged 4–6 years. [Abstracts issue – 10th Annual Conference of the International Society for Quality of Life Research.] Quality of Life Research 12(7):794

Fabry G, Cheng LX, Molenaers G 1994 Normal and abnormal torsional development in children. Clinics in Orthopedics and Related Research (302):22–26

Galli M, Crivellini M, Santambrogio GC et al 2001 Short-term effects of 'botulinum toxin A' as treatment for children with cerebral palsy: kinematic and kinetic aspects at the ankle joint. Functional Neurology 16(4):317–323

Ganley JV 1984 Corrective casting in infants. Clinics in Podiatry 1(3):501–516

Ganley JV 1987 Podopediatrics: the past, present, and future challenge. Journal of the American Podiatric Medical Association 77(8):393

Ganley JV 1991 The hopscotch position: a screening test. Journal of the American Podiatric Medical Association 81(3):136

Gupta A, Singh S, Patel P et al 2008 Evaluation of the utility of the Ponseti method of correction of clubfoot deformity in a developing nation. International Orthopedics 32(1):75–79

Haft GF, Walker CG, Craxford AD 2007 Early clubfoot recurrence after use of the Ponseti method in a New Zealand population. Journal of Bone and Joint Surgery – American Volume 89(3):487–493

Harris EJ, Vanore JV, Thomas JL et al 2004 Diagnosis and treatment of pediatric flatfoot. Journal of Foot and Ankle Surgery 43:341–373

Hemo Y, Macdessi SJ, Pierce RA et al 2006 Outcome of patients after Achilles tendon lengthening for treatment of idiopathic toe walking. Journal of Pediatric Orthopedics 26(3):336–340

Herzenberg JE, Smith JD, Paley D 1994 Correcting torsional deformities with Ilizarov's apparatus. Clinical Orthopedics and Related Research (302):36–41

Herzenberg JE, Radler C, Bor N 2002 Ponseti versus traditional methods of casting for idiopathic clubfoot. Journal of Pediatric Orthopedics 22(4):517–521

Kite JH 1967 Errors and complications in treating foot conditions in children. Clinical Orthopaedics and Related Research 53:31–38

Kumar SJ, MacEwen GD 1982 Torsional abnormalities in children's lower extremities. Orthopedic Clinics of North America 13(3):629–639

Landorf KB, Keenan AM 2000 Efficacy of foot orthoses: what does the literature tell us? Journal of the American Podiatric Medical Association 90(3):149

Losel S, Burgess-Milliron MJ, Micheli LJ et al 1996 A simplified technique for determining foot progression angle in children 4 to 16 years of age. Journal of Pediatric Orthopedics 16(5):570–574

Morcuende JA, Dolan LA, Dietz FR et al 2004 Radical reduction in the rate of extensive corrective surgery for clubfoot using the Ponseti method. Pediatrics 113(2):376–380

Morcuende JA, Abbasi D, Dolan LA et al 2005 Results of an accelerated Ponseti protocol for clubfoot. Journal of Pediatric Orthopedics 25(5):623–626

Pfeiffer M, Kotz R, Ledl T et al 2006 Prevalence of flat foot in preschool-aged children. Pediatrics 118(2):634–639

Ponseti IV, Morcuende JA, Mosca V et al 2003 Clubfoot: Ponseti management, 2nd edn. Global HELP Publication. Online. Available at: http://www.global-help.org/publications/books/book_cfponseti.html (accessed 4 May 2009)

Ponseti IV, Zhivkov M, Davis N et al 2006 Treatment of the complex idiopathic clubfoot. Clinical Orthopaedics and Related Research 451:171–176

Powell M, Seid M, Szer IS 2005 Efficacy of custom foot orthoses in improving pain and functional status in children with juvenile idiopathic arthritis: a randomized trial. Journal of Rheumatology 32(5):943–950

Rome K, Ashford RL, Evans AM 2006 Non-surgical interventions for paediatric pes planus. Cochrane Database of Systematic Reviews (4):1–7

Ruta DA, Garratt AM, Leng M et al 1994 A new approach to the measurement of quality of life: the patient-generated index. Medical Care 32:1109–1126

Staheli LT 1987 Evaluation of planovalgus foot deformities with special reference to the natural history. Journal of the American Podiatric Medical Association 77(1):2–6

Staheli LT 1999 Planovalgus foot deformity. Current status [see comments]. [Review] [28 refs]. Journal of the American Podiatric Medical Association 89(2):94–99

Thacker MM, Scher DM, Sala DM et al 2005 Use of the foot abduction orthosis following Ponseti casts: is it essential? Journal of Pediatric Orthopedics 25(2):225–228

Thackeray C, Beeson P 1996a Is in-toeing gait a developmental stage? The Foot 6:19–24

Thackeray C, Beeson P 1996b In-toeing gait in children: a review of the literature. The Foot 6:1–4

Valmassy RL 1996 Clinical biomechanics of the lower extremities. Mosby, St Louis, p. 246

Wenger DR, Mauldin D, Speck G et al 1989 Corrective shoes and inserts as treatment for flexible flatfoot in infants and children [see comments]. Journal of Bone and Joint Surgery – American Volume 71(6):800–810

Whitford D, Esterman A 2007 A randomized controlled trial of two types of in-shoe orthoses in children with flexible excess pronation of the feet. Foot and Ankle International 28(6):715–723

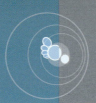

Glossary

Acetabular: pertaining to the pelvic hip joint 'cups' or sockets.

Active: cartilage to bone turnover region between diaphysis and epiphysis.

Adductus: adducted.

AFO: ankle foot orthosis.

Allodynia: painful response to light touch.

Amenorrhoea: absence of menstruation.

Ankle rocker: a three-phase model which describes the forward progression of the ankle in stance and relates range of motion, timing of muscle firing and coordinated strength.

Anlage: (cartilage) template or model (upon which bone forms).

Antetorsion: read: femoral torsion.

Anteversion: read: position of femur relative to hip joint.

Apophyses: epiphyses with a tendon attached.

Arch index: width of footprint arch/width of footprint heel; developed by Staheli.

Arthrogryposis: shortened term for arthrogryposis multiplex congenita (AMC) – congenital deformity of multiple joints.

Atavism: adduction of the hallux may function in gait as an adductory 'thumb': May contribute to intoeing gait pattern nullified with straight last footwear.

Avascular necrosis: tissue death due to insufficient blood supply.

Barlow's test: manual test for infant hip stability where the hips are abducted and the head of femur is (re)placed in the acetabulum.

Beighton scale: nine point scale for assessment of hypermobility.

Blount's disease: altered growth of the knee epiphysis resulting in increased genu varum.

Botox: botulinum toxin type A – a toxin which acts on the motor end plates by inhibiting the neurotransmitter acetylcholine.

Cadence: number of steps per unit time.

Calcaneovalgus: congenital foot position of abduction, eversion and foot (may be) dorsiflexed to touch the tibia; tightness of tibialis anterior is common.

Chondrification: cartilage development.

Chondroblasts: cells producing cartilage.

Chondroclasts: cells associated with cartilage resorption.

Coalition: joining of two bones by an intervening 'bridge'.

Concentric: muscle loading, contraction with decreased length.

Corpus callosum: white matter of the brain joining the two cerebral hemispheres.

Coxa valga: angle greater than 90° between femoral head/neck and the femoral shaft in the frontal/coronal plane associated with genu varum.

Coxa vara: angle less than 90° between femoral head/neck and the femoral shaft in the frontal/coronal plane associated with genu valgum.

DAFO: dynamic ankle foot orthosis.

Denis Browne bar: traditional orthopaedic torsion splint.

Diaphysis: central shaft of a long bone.

Dimeglio: alternative scoring system for clubfoot severity. Useful for walking children as gait parameters are included.

Diplegia: spasticity affecting both legs.

Dorsiflexion: flexion of the ankle in the sagittal plane.

Eccentric: muscle loading, contraction with increased length.

Ectoderm: outer layer from zygote division differentiates to form skin, nerves.

Ekbom's syndrome: usually called restless legs syndrome. Dr Karl Ekbom identified and named this condition.

Embryo: conceived 'body' within the first 8 weeks of gestation.

Embryonic: pertaining to the first 8 weeks of gestation.

Endochondral ossification: the process of bone formation from a cartilage template.

Endoderm: inner layer from zygote division differentiates to form gastrointestinal, respiratory linings.

Epiphyses: secondary centre of ossification. Separated from the metaphysis by the epiphyseal plate.

Equino: equine – horse, plantarflexed attitude.

Equinus: plantarflexion (extension) of the foot on the leg.

ESR: erythrocyte sedimentation rate elevation indicates increased immune response, e.g. infection.

EVA: ethylene vinyl acetate.

Fetus: the matured embryo, i.e. from week 8 to birth.

Genicular: refers to the knee.

Greenstick fracture: incomplete fracture type occurring in young bone. Only one side of the diaphyseal shaft cortex is disrupted, so the bone bends without breaking, as occurs when a green stick is bent.

Haemophilia: hereditary blood disorder of reduced/absent blood plasma clotting factors associated with haemorrhages.

Hemiplegia: cerebral palsy affecting one side of the body, i.e. one arm and one leg.

HPV: human papilloma virus.

Hyaline cartilage: covers articular joint surfaces.

Hydrocephalus: 'water on the brain' – abnormal and enlarged skull formation due to excess cerebrospinal fluid.

Hypermobility: increased joint range.

Hypertonia: high muscle tone, rigid feel to muscle bellies.

Hypertonic: increased (muscle) tone.

Hypertonicity: increased muscle tone (excitation).

Hypotonia: low muscle tone, flaccid feel to muscle bellies, associated with 'floppy baby' condition.

Hypoxia: lack of adequate oxygen.

Idiopathic: condition of unknown cause.

Jack's test: dorsiflexion of the hallux of the weight-bearing foot indicative of the efficiency of the plantar fascial windlass mechanism.

Keratinocytes: cells which produce skin keratin.

Kinematic: the angular, spatial component of gait/motion analysis.

Kinetic: the forces associated with gait/motion analysis.

Kyphosis: forward bend (of the spine) in the sagittal plane. Typically thoracic.

Kyphotic: forward curve (of the spine) in the sagittal plane – 'hump back'.

Lordosis: backward bend (of the spine) in the sagittal plane – 'hollow back'. Opposite curve of kyphosis. Typically lumbar spine.

Mesenchyme: derived from mesoderm, the middle layer of differentiated zygote tissue, forms bones, muscle, connective tissues, blood.

Mesoderm: middle layer from zygote division, differentiates to form bones, muscle, connective tissues, blood.

Metaphysis: vascular region of bone at either end of the diaphysis.

Metatarsus: metatarsals.

Metatarsus adductus: metatarsals adducted from the tarso-metatarso (Lisfranc) joint relative to the rear foot.

Metatarsus primus varus: the first ray has an adducted and varus position, the intermetatarsal angle is increased, concave medial foot border, straight lateral border.

Metatarsus varus: metatarsals are adducted and varus from Lisfranc joint, commonly a synonym for metatarsus adductus.

Mg: magnesium.

Mitchell bar: new torsion splint developed specifically for use with the Ponseti method.

Monofilament: Semmes-Weinstein monofilament graded by the load required to optically flex the filament; clinically 1 g, 5 g, 10 g are commonly used.

Morphology: shape and form.

Morton's foot: characterized by a short first ray and the appearance of a long second toe (relatively). Identified and named by Dr Alex Morton.

Myelomeningocele: herniation of meninges containing part of the spinal cord.

Neoplasm: new growth.

Neural tension: tightness of lower limb nerve, a common source of pain.

Oligohydramnios: insufficient amniotic fluid during pregnancy.

Orthoses: from the Greek *orthos*, meaning to straighten.

Ortolani's test: manual test for infant hip stability where the hips are adducted and loaded posteriorly to see if subluxation or dislocation occur.

Ossification: process of bone formation.

Osteoblasts: cells producing bone.

Osteoclasts: cells associated with bone resorption.

Pathognomonic: specifically defining, e.g. talipes equinovarus and equinus.

Pedotopography: photography of the weight-bearing surface of the foot.

Periosteal: pertaining to the 'skin' covering of bones.

Periostitis: inflammation of the periosteum (bone 'skin').

Pes cavus: high arched, supinated foot type; suggestive of neurological problem; Charcot–Marie–Tooth, Friedrich's ataxia, peroneal muscle atrophy are common associations.

Physeal: pertaining to physis.

Physis: 'growth plate'.

Pirani: refers to Dr Sharif Pirani, colleague of Dr Ponseti; invented a six point clubfoot scoring system.

Plagiocephaly: flattening and misshaping of the infant head due to prolonged forces in one position.

Plantarflexion: extension of the ankle in the sagittal plane.

Ponseti: refers to Dr Ignacio Ponseti, orthopaedic surgeon, who invented the non-surgical Ponseti method for management of infant clubfoot.

Ponseti method: non-surgical method of clubfoot correction.

Pronated: opposite of supination, triplane position: abduction, eversion, dorsiflexion.

Recurvatum: hyperextension of a (knee) joint posteriorly.

Reliability: repeatability of measures.
  Intra-rater reliability: repeated measures of an individual examiner – only relevant to the individual examiner.
  Inter-rater reliability: repeated measures between different examiners – relevant to all examiners.

Rete ridge: the parallel lines seen within the epidermis parallel pattern is interrupted by verrucae, lines deviate.

Root model: model of foot biomechanics from the 1970s developed by podiatrists Merton Root, John Weed, Bill Orien.

Rydel Seiffer: a quantitative tuning fork (128 Hz) scaled from 0–8 octals.

S1–S2: denotes the junction of the first and second sacral vertebrae.

Salter–Harris: classification system for epiphyseal plate injuries.

Seronegative: autoimmune, inflammatory conditions. Pertains to the negative blood markers.

SFS: stabilizing foot splint; customized non-cast thermoplastic heel cup device.

Spastic: high tone muscles which 'spasm' and give rise to 'spastic' motion.

Steenbeck bar: torsion splint developed in Uganda for post casting maintenance.

Supernumerary: in addition to the usual number found. May be a synonymous term with 'accessory'.

Supinated: triplane position: adduction, inversion, plantarflexion.

Synchondrosis: cartilage coalition.

Syndesmosis: fibrous coalition.

Synostosis: osseous coalition.

Talipes: deformity of the foot; tali – talus (ankle), pes – foot.

Teratogens: introduced toxins which deleteriously alter fetal development.

TEV: talipes equinovarus.

Thermoplastic: material which deforms with heat and sets with cooling.

Thrombosis: blood clotting, blocking vessel patency.

Tibial plafond: distal end of tibia surface which approximates the transverse plane and opposes the talar trochlear surface; part of the ankle joint.

Transmalleolar axis: the line formed by joining the fibular and tibial malleoli often used as a proxy for tibial torsion (fraught, as the proximal tibia and distal tibia fibula are compared).

Triceps surae: calf muscle group, gastrocnemius and soleus.

Trimester: three months of pregnancy.

Triplane wedge: an in-shoe version of the cobbler's Thomas heel promoted by podiatrist Ron Valmassy; originally comprised a heel wedge to invert/dorsiflex the calcaneus.

UCBL: University of California Biomechanics Laboratory. Refers to a high cupped and flanged foot orthosis.

USAGPQ: University of South Australia Growing Pains Questionnaire (Appendix 7.1).

Varus: inverted in the frontal/coronal plane.

Young's modulus: of elasticity: the ratio between stress and strain.

Zn: zinc.

Zygote: embryonic cell mass.

Index

N.B. Page numbers in *italic* denote figures or tables.

B.b. # 573695

618.927
EVA